Selecting and Implementing Evidence-Based Practice

Rosalyn Bertram · Suzanne Kerns

Selecting and Implementing Evidence-Based Practice

A Practical Program Guide

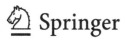 Springer

Rosalyn Bertram, Ph.D.
Professor
School of Social Work
University of Missouri–Kansas City
Kansas City, MO, USA

Suzanne Kerns, Ph.D.
Research Associate Professor
Graduate School of Social Work
University of Denver
Denver, CO, USA

ISBN 978-3-030-11324-7   ISBN 978-3-030-11325-4   (eBook)
https://doi.org/10.1007/978-3-030-11325-4

Library of Congress Control Number: 2019933388

This Springer imprint is published by the registered company Springer Nature Switzerland AG
The registered company address is: Gewerbestrasse 11, 6330 Cham, Switzerland

Foreword

After reading this well-written manuscript, my reaction was one of great appreciation to the authors for reminding the field that the scientist–practitioner model is not dead and is totally attainable and more important than ever for the provision of effective behavioral health care. The authors, both true exemplars of this model, have presented a clear, well-documented account of the background and current status of the use of evidence-based practice in the broad mental health field. I think this book will serve as a valuable resource for clinicians, administrators, students, faculty, and academicians. I would also recommend it to family organizations as a resource in their education programs for the families they serve. Families with children who are experiencing emotional and behavioral challenges must understand the critical need to obtain the most effective treatment available for their child. Why waste precious time on methods that do not work?

Bertram and Kerns have done an excellent job of blending hard science, clinical applications, and big picture issues into a very readable volume that will have valuable information for the diverse audiences mentioned above. They confront readers with some hard facts. We are living in a time of anti-intellectualism and antiscience that has been justifiably compared to ancient eras. However, they bring home a very tangible and current result of this by noting that only 1 in 10 persons receiving behavioral treatment today are receiving an evidence-based practice. I hope that this will rally readers to examine their own practice and become advocates for change in this dismal situation.

A strength of the book is its organization and flow of information. As I read it, I thought of the different hats I have worn in my career: clinician, faculty member, researcher, program developer, and parent. Typically, a text will present material that will focus on one of those hats. In this text, Bertram and Kerns skillfully present material in a balanced fashion that will keep the attention of a diverse audience throughout the pages. Obviously, there are sections that are aimed at specific groups. Chapters 5 and 8 will appeal to faculty and program developers and administrators, but they are presented in a way that a clinician, whether new or seasoned, will appreciate the challenge-facing workforce developers. In these chapters, the authors have given us hope for the future. There are places that have begun the process of curriculum improvement, and readers can use this information as a resource for their own efforts. Other chapters are clearly more universal with their content. Everyone needs to understand the terminology. The presentation in Chap. 3 gives a good historical perspective on the field and the debates that emerged. Beginning in this chapter and continuing in Chap. 4 on myths, I was impressed by the fair presentation of the controversial issues that challenge evidence-based practice. These issues have been hotly debated, and it is easy to skim some points to support your own biases. Bertram and Kerns have skillfully avoided this.

I think Chaps. 6–11 provide a core of knowledge that is critical for anyone who is a practitioner. There are very few resources to my knowledge that explain the extreme importance of the underlying components of evidence-based practice. Regardless of your role in the field, it is of the utmost necessity to be totally proficient in the value of treatment fidelity and documenting it, as well as in data-based decision making and the principles of implementation science. Sadly, these topics rarely receive the depth of explication that Bertram and Kerns present, and this contributes to the value of this book.

Chapter 12 is a bonus for readers. The experience and hard work of the authors are put to use in their presentation of very practical information. They go beyond theory and tackle the tough issues of curriculum reform, funding, insurance, and even offer suggestions for faculty grant writing based on the integration of the information in the preceding chapters—an excellent conclusion to a fact-based, clearly presented text.

Albert Duchnowski, Ph.D.
Professor Emeritus
University of South Florida
Tampa, Florida

Acknowledgements

We wish to acknowledge Dr. Bertram's graduate research assistant, Soo-Whan Choi, M.A., who provided significant support in the edits and organization of this book.

We extend our thanks to Katherine Briar-Lawson, Ph.D., LMSW, Professor and Dean Emeritus at the School of Social Welfare, University at Albany, SUNY, and the National Child Welfare Workforce Institute; to Al Duchnowski Ph.D., Professor Emeritus at the Department of Child and Family Studies, College of Behavioral and Community Sciences, University of South Florida; and to Virginia Strand, Ph.D. Professor, Fordham University Graduate School of Social Service, for their careful reviews and suggestions.

In developing this book, we drew on myriad examples from our professional work. We acknowledge our community and academic collaborators who shaped and shared our collective journey of learning. Finally, we deeply appreciate our partners and families for their love, understanding, and support through the many long days, late nights, and busy weekends spent in our research and writing.

Contents

Chapter 1
Beginning with the End in Mind

We are experiencing an unusual moment in history. The scientific method which has produced health care and technological innovations that extend lives and instantaneously connect us across vast distance is being ignored, minimized, and undermined when proven facts are deemed inconvenient. Myths, misconceptions, propaganda, and ideology are passionately asserted to challenge science when findings suggest a new and necessary path that will disrupt accustomed practice and belief. In this, through the looking glass moment, opinion or faith are asserted as alternative facts to avert inconvenient truths.

Sadly, such perspectives are not limited to the political perturbations of this historical period in some democracies. For two decades, behavioral health care, social services, and academic programs have struggled to understand and embrace, to provide and to teach the selection and implementation of evidence-based practice. How can this be? We expect our veterinarian to treat our beloved pets with the most proven practice. We expect the same from our dentist, our gynecologist, and family physician. Are social services and behavioral health care somehow intrinsically different? We think not.

This book is intended for use by both academic and behavioral health care programs. We identify the content and processes to improve workforce preparation and behavioral health care service provision. Our premises are simple. Evidence-based practice is logical and, when well implemented, is effective and sustainable. Eclectic practice is neither proven nor sustainable. Sound research can easily be explored to identify effective practices that, if well implemented, can be sustained to improve consumer outcomes in less time and at less cost.

Chapter 3 presents a brief history of the emergence of evidence-based practice from the field of medicine in the 1990s. We discuss confusion and debates about definitional criteria, as well as values and theory bias in common critiques of evidence-based practice made by social service and behavioral health professions. We believe there is an evidence-informed process in the work of good doctors and good social service and behavioral health care practitioners, and each profession applies specific evidence-based practices. We address the unfortunate and unnecessary perception that there are significant differences between proponents of a ***process of evidence-***

© Springer Nature Switzerland AG 2019
R. Bertram and S. Kerns, *Selecting and Implementing Evidence-Based Practice*,
https://doi.org/10.1007/978-3-030-11325-4_1

based practice and advocates for specific *evidence-based practice models* while clarifying confusion generated by a plethora of terms, myths, and misperceptions. We assert it is long past time for debate, as Chap. 4 addresses the most common myths and misconceptions with facts.

Chapter 5 explores academic workforce preparation, the influence of curricula and the development of knowledge and skills necessary for evidence-based practice. Tapping research conducted by participants in the Child and Family Evidence-Based Practice Consortium, this chapter helps faculty and students to anticipate challenges to curricula transformation. We present the perspectives of program deans, chairs, and directors who identified faculty knowledge and beliefs as a primary barrier to integrating evidence-based practice in the curriculum (Bertram, Charnin, Kerns, & Long, 2015). Responses from these academic leaders also include how teaching evidence-based practice and implementation science can enhance the academic program's reputation, attracting students and faculty who want to work with service organizations to fund the selection and implementation of evidence-based practices. Academic leaders also describe the graduates of these programs as feeling more competent and confident, knowing they have developed current and marketable knowledge and skills.

Chapter 6 presents how an innovative program establishes itself as a promising practice first in efficacy trials and then establishes itself as an evidence-based practice in studies of effectiveness and dissemination. We highlight the importance of developing practical measures of fidelity and written guidelines identifying key elements and activities that contribute to improved client outcomes. These guidelines also serve as a map for negotiating treatment challenges with clients.

Chapter 7 identifies evidence-based practices that address common behavioral health problems such as anxiety, depression, traumatic stress, and child behavioral health concerns. We highlight common elements and conclude with an example of how a strategic set of evidence-based practices could provide a continuum of services to address the majority of a community's behavioral health concerns for children, youth, and families.

Chapter 8 introduces implementation science, which provides blueprints for installation of a selected evidence-based practice. We present frameworks identified by the National Implementation Research Network's seminal study of over 800 empirical studies and meta-analyses of effective implementation efforts in a wide variety of settings and endeavors (Fixsen, Naoom, Blase, Friedman, & Wallace, 2005). We also review Damschroder's framework for implementation (Damschroder et al. 2009) as well as practical approaches informed by Powell and colleagues' taxonomy of implementation support strategies (Powell et al., 2015). We emphasize that slowing down to align agency infrastructure with a new practice, and carefully considering strategies for its successful implementation, is time well spent. Based on community culture and organizational context, we also discuss the "adaptable periphery"of a practice that can and might need to be adjusted.

Chapter 9 emphasizes the importance of beginning initial implementation in a transformation zone to enact readiness activities, training, and best practices for on-the-job workforce development. We highlight the importance of behavioral rehearsal as a key approach to knowledge transfer and explore different supervision and consultation approaches that support delivery of an evidence-based practice with fidelity.

Chapter 10 discusses practical challenges often experienced during initial implementation of an evidence-based practice. We offer strategies to anticipate and hopefully avoid them, as well as how to learn from and address them when they do arise. For example, it is common for practitioners to initially struggle with the elements and activities of a new intervention as they use it with clients. This struggle is normal but can perpetuate the myth that evidence-based practices are "cookie cutter" and leave little room for practitioner creativity and style. We discuss how to conceptualize the stage of initial implementation in a way that mitigates the risk of such erroneous attributions.

Chapter 11 presents how data should inform selection and implementation of an evidence-based practice. This includes the use of implementation teams as well as monitoring practice fidelity and the alignment of implementation drivers that support the organization's ability to improve client outcomes. First, we explore the use of data to inform the selection of evidence-based practice to address a particular need within a community. We review models such as Partnerships for Success and Getting to Outcomes and present examples illustrating how data guide community and organization decision making. We then describe approaches to inform the clinical process of implementation. Clinical feedback systems that monitor both symptoms and model fidelity now readily provide data that inform and guide decisions to improve outcomes. This discussion includes the use of the EBP toolkit and PracticeWise clinical dashboard.

Finally, in Chap. 12, we suggest future program pathways. With only 1 in 10 people receiving an intervention that could be considered evidence-based, there is a long road ahead before we achieve population-level saturation of effective practices. In this final chapter, through allegory and through current examples, we explore how academic programs can integrate evidence-based practice and implementation science into courses and field curricula, while collaborating with behavioral health or social service programs to do so.

Funding sources and health insurance providers increasingly require the use of effective practices. Administrators, supervisors, and practitioners must be comfortable with finding and critically examining the strength of evidence for particular practices, and be well versed in their effective implementation. Teaching students how to critically examine research supporting evidence-based practices, as well as how to implement and evaluate these practices, aligns an academic program with major funding sources and with the needs of the organizations that hire its graduates. In the final chapter, we discuss how adjusting curricula in this manner offers faculty pathways to securing grants and contracts to conduct applied research, to provide technical assistance, and to conduct program implementation evaluations that offer multiple publishing opportunities.

References

Bertram, R. M., Charnin, L. A., Kerns, S. E. U., & Long, A. C. (2015). Evidence-based practices in North American MSW curricula. *Research on Social Work Practice, 25*(6), 737–748.

Damschroder, L. J., Aron, D. C., Keith, R. E., Kirsh, S. R., Alexander, J. A., & Lowery, J. C. (2009). Fostering implementation of health services research findings into practice: A consolidated framework for advancing implementation science. *Implementation science, 4*(1), 50.

Fixsen, D. L., Naoom, S. F., Blase, K. A., Friedman, R. M., & Wallace, F. (2005). *Implementation research: A synthesis of the literature*. Tampa, FL: University of South Florida, Louis de la Parte Florida Mental Health Institute, The National Implementation Research Network (FMHI Publication #231).

Powell, B. J., Waltz, T. J., Chinman, M. J., Damschroder, L. J., Smith, J. L., Matthieu, M. M., … & Kirchner, J. E. (2015). A refined compilation of implementation strategies: Results from the Expert Recommendations for Implementing Change (ERIC) project. *Implementation Science, 10*(1), 21.

Chapter 2
Visiting the Clinic:
A Child and Family Tale

We begin with a story about Tameisha's family, school, and community. As you read, observe how different people try to understand and to address this situation. Consider how this situation might be addressed in the community where you grew up or where you now work and live. Would the story have a similar ending? Why or why not?

Once upon a time, a twelve-year-old African-American girl named Tameisha was not well. She seemed tired and detached, perhaps even sad. As recently as a year and a half ago, she was an excellent student and athlete, eagerly completing assigned readings and focusing for hours how best to compose written assignments. When this work was complete, she joined friends from her school and church to gleefully play their favorite sports. She would return home to devour dinner and discuss her friends and classes with her parents and younger brother. She sang in the community church's choir where her father served as a deacon and most of her friends and their families also worshiped. Her extended family also participated in this church and on Sundays would gather for family dinner and conversation. Life was good. While both of her parents worked hard at their jobs, they spent a great amount of time together as a family. They enjoyed vacations to southern states and the Caribbean to visit relatives and track some of their origins.

Recently Tameisha's zest for life had diminished. Just before their last vacation, her father had been downsized from his job. A new position was secured but required a long commute. The family moved midway between her mother's place of employment and father's new workplace into a mixed race, but primarily Euro-American community. As a new African-American student, Tameisha stood out. Taunted for her interest in history, her timely submission of assignments, and her joy in sports, she began to complain of vague physical maladies and frequently missed classes while visiting the nurse's office. Over time, her academic performance deteriorated. She was placed in remedial courses with disruptive students who demonstrated anti-social behaviors in class, on the school playground, and in the community. These

© Springer Nature Switzerland AG 2019   5
R. Bertram and S. Kerns, *Selecting and Implementing Evidence-Based Practice*,
https://doi.org/10.1007/978-3-030-11325-4_2

students also taunted her interest in sports, attributing it to her racial background, and she eventually withdrew from sporting activities. Her fearsome appetite for food, friendship, and knowledge became a fading shadow of its former self. She ate little and spoke even less.

Tameisha's parents sought medical help at the local clinic where, with the family, the nurse explored the history of this unexpected behavior change. They sought to identify the last time the young girl was more her active self. But, time and emergence of behaviors can be difficult to pinpoint amidst significant contextual change. Was it before or after the last vacation? Was it before or after her father lost his job? Or was it when he began the long commutes to his new workplace? Her behaviors definitely worsened when the family moved to a new community and school district.

Although Tameisha was quite apprehensive about meeting the doctor, her parents reassured that this practitioner was well-trained, from the best of schools, active in research, and quite knowledgeable about child development. The doctor examined the literature from several studies addressing symptoms of decreased appetite and listlessness. Seeking to rule out any physical anomalies, the doctor ran a series of medically suggested tests that examined blood, metabolism, bone structure, heart, and lung capacity. The tests suggested changes in digestive capacity, prompting an imaging of the digestive tract, where a parasite was found. Perhaps, it was from food eaten on that vacation immediately before the family experienced changes of job, residence, and school. After examining *Cochrane systematic reviews*, the doctor recommended a specific diet change concurrent with the medication most likely to eliminate the parasite.

Initiated in 1992, the Cochrane Collaboration (www.cochrane.org) *is dedicated to publishing systematic reviews of primary healthcare research. Named after the British epidemiologist Archie Cochrane, this essential tool for assessment and intervention was first established to evaluate available evidence from randomized controlled trials. Its underlying assumption is that health care interventions will be more effective if they are based on complete, current, and reliable evidence instead of dated research, anecdote, and conjecture. Updated regularly, the reviews now examine effects of interventions as well as the accuracy of diagnostic tests for specific conditions, patient groups, and settings.*

However, the doctor noted there were a significant number of disruptions in the family's accustomed activities and recommended that if the medical intervention did not help improve the girl's behavior, the family should seek help at a behavioral healthcare clinic. When the family balked at the thought of seeking counseling at a mental health center, the doctor suggested they work closely with school personnel.

The medicine eliminated the parasite, but Tameisha remained averse to academic and sports activities as the taunts and teasing by her peers continued. Although she complained to her teacher and to the school counselor, she saw no actions taken by the school to address the incessant racially tinged bullying. The only action that diminished the teasing was when she joined those bullying students in disrupting the remedial classes.

Her parents met with a child study team that included the school social worker, psychologist, and the girl's teachers. The child study team was entirely focused on current grades and behaviors. There was no meaningful exploration of Tameisha's grades, behaviors, and social activities at her previous school. Some on the study team seemed to attribute the change in performance and behavior to the onset of adolescence. The psychologist recommended a battery of personality and intelligence tests that ultimately suggested anxiety and depression obscuring high intelligence. Nevertheless, in hopes that Tameisha would become more academically engaged, the teachers developed less challenging lesson plans, ostensibly to facilitate success. However, the lowered expectations in assignments were boring and the frequency of her disruptive behaviors increased.

As a result, the school social worker was directed to provide individual counseling whenever Tameisha disrupted the classroom. The counseling removed her from class but did not consistently provide any proven treatment. The school social worker used techniques he learned at workshops for building a therapeutic relationship. One of those continuing education workshops presented Motivational Interviewing, an evidence-based practice developed for motivating substance using clients to change behaviors. As in most school districts, there was no regularly scheduled supervision, so the social worker received no coaching on his use of Motivational Interviewing. As time passed and Tameisha's disruptive behavior continued, he altered treatment to a psychodynamic exploration of her depression. He combined this with what he believed was a behavioral approach, rewarding her with a lunch treat when she was not sent to his office. When this was not productive, he increasingly used a quiet time procedure to help Tameisha calm down to return to class. The family was not engaged in the counseling, and no other proven practice was delivered in the months of continued disruptive behavior.

Because there was no improvement, the school threatened suspension, so despite the family's aversion to seeking help at what they perceived as a psychiatric center, the parents took their daughter to the behavioral healthcare clinic recommended by their doctor. Unlike the school services, this clinic provided only family-centered evidence-based practices. An intake specialist developed a behavioral history with the family similar to that conducted by the nurse in the medical clinic. Based upon the behaviors and the change of jobs, homes, schools, and community, a practitioner trained and supervised in Multisystemic Therapy (MST) was introduced who arranged to meet the family at their home in the evening after both parents returned from work.

> *MST is an **evidence-based practice model** proven effective for addressing anti-social youth behaviors with over two decades of random assignment control group studies* (Hengeller et al., 2009). *Based in ecological systems theory, its protocol, training, coaching, and use of data to maintain fidelity and achieve client outcomes are well-tested through multiple random controlled studies in a variety of settings with different client populations and behaviors of concern.*

They discussed the parents' and Tameisha's concerns and established overarching goals for their work together. Not surprisingly the family shared a desire to see their daughter return to her previous excellent academic performance and for her to have friends who shared her interests in sports.

Following MST protocol, the clinician engaged the mother, the father, and their daughter in an exploration of what they thought contributed to Tameisha's academic and social well-being at her previous school before the family moved. The clinician pursued their perspectives about contributing factors in the youth, her peers, her school, in their family and community. Following MST protocol, they drew these factors in an ecological fit circle assessment that identified which contributing factors seemed most proximal or pertinent to the girls' previous strong academic performance and social well-being. It was evident that prior to the change in residence, the parents were better able to monitor their daughter's interests, friends, and activities because extended family and church members naturally observed and shared their knowledge of Tameisha and her friends.

The clinician and family then shifted their assessment to focus upon the girl's current disruptive classroom behaviors and diminished interests in sports and other pro-social activities since the family moved to a new school district. They discussed and identified possible contributing factors in the youth, her peers, in the family, in the school, and in the community. This residence change moved the family away from church and extended family supports. It exposed Tameisha to racial taunts from antisocial peers that school authorities failed to address. These appeared to be the proximal contributing factors to Tameisha's antisocial behaviors and poor academic performance.

Through this thorough ecological assessment, it was easy to see that before the family moved, the parents more closely monitored and encouraged Tameisha's academic and sports activities. They knew who her friends were, and at dinner each night would discuss what she and her friends were thinking and doing in class assignments and in the sports activities. It was just as obvious that since the change of residence and schools, the parents did not know their daughter's friends or acquaintances that school interventions were not addressing the teasing and taunts and that some school interventions actually contributed to Tameisha's listlessness by not challenging her in class assignments. Tameisha freely stated she disrupted class to escape boredom with the teachers' new assignments and to escape the bullying and teasing. She also shared that counseling by the school social worker was not helpful because he was always trying to motivate her to develop insight about her depression.

Together with the MST clinician, the family designed and implemented interventions to improve parental monitoring and coaching their daughter on how to negotiate taunts from classmates. Each intervention was evaluated by the family with the MST practitioner, and lessons learned were added to their ecological assessment.

They also agreed there must be more active monitoring of school interventions. This required exchanging information with school personnel several times each week about Tameisha's classroom behavior and its relationship with peer taunts and teasing. With this data, another intervention built upon the father's leadership abilities that were previously manifest in his role as a church deacon. He insisted on a face-to-face meeting with school administrators to directly address the racial taunts and bullying. Teachers were eventually included in these discussions that produced a more proactive intervention in which Tameisha could signal the teacher when she was being taunted and the teacher would immediately assign her a task in the school library where she worked on more challenging academic assignments. As her behavior and grades improved, the school allowed Tameisha to participate in her favorite sports where she began developing pro-social peer relationships. Within four months the family had achieved their goals and by inviting their daughter's new pro-social friends and their parents to a backyard barbeque, the parents began developing social supports in their new community.

Eclectic or Evidence-Based Practice?

In this child and family tale, using techniques learned in continuing education workshops, the school social worker applied an eclectic approach to try to establish a therapeutic relationship with the girl. These workshops emphasized that the practitioner—client relationship was the basis for improving outcomes as the practitioner applies professional knowledge and skills in an eclectic creative selection of interventions individualized for each client. One of the continuing education workshops presented Motivational Interviewing, an evidence-based practice developed for motivating substance using clients to change behaviors. However, as in most school settings, there was no regularly scheduled formal supervision, and the social worker received no coaching on consistent adherence (fidelity) to Motivational Interviewing. With no appreciable academic or behavioral improvement, the school social worker shifted to using psychodynamic counseling techniques to help Tameisha develop insight into her depression which he believed was the source of her academic struggles and behaviors. When she was not sent to his office, he used contingency reinforcement, offering lunch treats. When this eclectic mix of interventions was not effective, his counseling with Tameisha primarily provided quiet time, so she could calm down and return to class.

When the school interventions did not meaningfully improve Tameisha's academic performance or behavior, the family engaged an MST practitioner who visited their home at times of their convenience several days a week. The MST practitioner explained why MST would work for this family, and that it had been specifically developed and tested in multiple experimental studies to effectively address disruptive or antisocial youth behavior. The MST practitioner worked within written guidelines that were refined and proven effective in those studies. With Tameisha and her family, each activity or element was individualized so that the ecological assessment and interventions applied family-identified strengths to address contributing factors that maintained the poor academic performance and the behaviors of concern. Each week, the MST practitioner submitted a case-specific assessment, planning, and intervention data to her supervisor who shared it with an MST consultant. From these data, and similar data submitted by other MST practitioners working with other families, the consultant and supervisor developed a focus and format for coaching the practitioners so their MST knowledge and skills improved and their clients' desired outcomes were achieved.

The most compelling reason for implementing evidence-based behavioral health practices is that they are more likely to improve client outcomes than unproven interventions (Weisz, Eckshtain, Ugueto, Hawley, & Jensen-Doss, 2013). In our allegorical child and family tale, the doctor at the medical clinic engaged the family in a thorough ecological assessment process that guided a search for and selection of proven practices that efficiently addressed the medical concern. The doctor noted there were a significant number of disruptions in the family's accustomed activities and supports and recommended that if the medical intervention did not help improve Tameisha's behavior, the family should seek help at a family-centered behavioral healthcare clinic.

The school personnel used traditional child-centered assessment. Their interventions focused directly on the symptoms of diminished academic performance and disruptive behavior in the school setting. Their assessments and interventions did not engage the parents and actually exacerbated the academic and behavioral concerns.

However, like the doctor, the MST practitioner explored ecological factors that might contribute to Tameisha's diminished academic performance and disruptive behavior. Unlike school personnel, the MST practitioner engaged the parents with their daughter in assessments and interventions while working within theory-based principles of a practice model proven effective in addressing such behaviors. Also, unlike school personnel, the MST clinician was well supported by data-informed, regularly scheduled, model-pertinent coaching.

The school social worker and MST practitioner graduated from Masters of Social Work (MSW) programs where they learned social work values and ethics and were exposed to a variety of theories and techniques to identify and address client needs. The school social worker received no on the job training in proven practice models, but was encouraged to pursue continuing education workshops of his choosing as he worked to earn clinical licensure.

In contrast, after a careful hiring process designed to evaluate whether she could work within a data-informed process of coaching, the MST practitioner immediately received five days of training about the population she would be working with as well as the theory-based and well-proven principles and processes of MST assessment, planning, intervention, and evaluation. She worked with three other MST practitioners who all received coaching from a supervisor who reviewed case data forms each week with an MST consultant who coached the supervisor in how best to improve each practitioner's MST knowledge and skills to apply MST with fidelity while achieving family goals.

Concerned about costs, school administrators chose to rely upon the academic preparation and continuing education pursued by its social worker to inform his clinical decisions. However, his MSW program did not teach a *process of evidence-based practice*. Behavioral health clinic administrators initially balked at costs to train practitioners and supervisors in MST and its use of model-pertinent data that informed consultation, supervision, and practice. However, they examined longitudinal cost-benefit analyses and concluded that by adopting MST, the clinic would have greater client and community impact while addressing funders' emphasis on improved outcomes and evidence-based practice.

As evidence-based practice became a subject of debate in social work and related disciplines, there was an inherent tension between proponents of eclectic practice and proponents of evidence-based practice. This discourse produced a plethora of definitions, criteria, and terms that fundamentally centered around the questions of whether evidence-based practice described a process of practice or whether it described specific treatment models. In the next chapter, we will examine these debates from the first decade of the twenty-first century, as well as their resolution.

Reference

Weisz, J. R., Kuppens, S., Eckshtain, D., Ugueto, A. M., Hawley, K. M., & Jensen-Doss, A. (2013). Performance of evidence-based youth psychotherapies compared with usual clinical care: A multilevel meta-analysis. *JAMA Psychiatry, 70,* 750–761.

Chapter 3
Definitions and Debates

Does the term *evidence-based practice* describe delivery of a treatment model that has been proven effective? Or, does the term describe a process of client engagement, assessment, selection, and delivery of interventions that are proven effective? Can both descriptions be true? What types of studies and how many studies are needed to warrant describing interventions or practice models as evidence-based? Does the term evidence-based imply that the practice works equally well across different populations? Can it be evidence-based if it was tested with a more limited demographic?

Initial debates in social work and related fields emerged from the chrysalis of these questions. Within the debates, strong assertions of opinion and belief too often overlooked or obscured facts about the implementation of evidence-based practice. Misperceptions and concerns emerged about the importance of practitioner creativity and expertise, and the practitioner–client relationship, as well as concerns about the responsibilities and resources of organizations.

In the previous chapter, both the school social worker and MST practitioner graduated from MSW programs that did not teach evidence-based practice. We shall see in Chap. 5, this is not unusual. For too long social work and related disciplines have debated whether or not evidence-based practice should be taught, and if taught, whether to teach a process for practice or specific treatment models or both. Rationale presented in these debates often reflected misperceptions and opinions that ignored or overlooked facts about evidence-based practice. In Chap. 4, we will address myths and common misconceptions with facts.

Confusing Definitions

In debates about evidence-based practice, well-meaning attempts to define it produced a plethora of terms that contributed to confusion and uncertainty. For example, to describe *specific treatment models*, some suggested using terms such as evidence-based practice, evidence-based treatment, research-based interventions, evidence-informed practice, and others. Suggested criteria for the amounts and types

© Springer Nature Switzerland AG 2019
R. Bertram and S. Kerns, *Selecting and Implementing Evidence-Based Practice*,
https://doi.org/10.1007/978-3-030-11325-4_3

of evidence for the terms varied or were often not even discussed. In describing *a process of practice*, some suggested using similar terms. These included evidence-based practice, research-based practice, and evidence-informed practice. Process descriptions included steps, essential elements, participants, and activities, but not criteria for the amount or types of evidence. These varying definitions caused a good degree of confusion.

For example, Thyer and Myers (2011) asserted evidence-based practice is a process of inquiry to help practitioners and their clients make decisions about service selection. They broadly declared there was no such thing as evidence-based practices, since the process of evidence-based practice considers research evidence, client preferences, values, and circumstance, as well as professional ethics, practitioner skills, and available resources. They asserted that evidence-based practice was not a noun, but a verb, and that interventions or techniques may be labeled as empirically supported or research-supported.

These early debates tended to describe social workers as though they were independent practitioners. This overlooked or ignored that most social workers are employed in service organizations, and that little by little, these organizations were adopting proven practice models. Early debates about defining evidence-based practice also did not address the emergence of implementation science, its clarification of the components of practice models, as well as how organizations must adjust to implement them effectively and with fidelity (Fixsen, Naoom, Blase, Friedman, & Wallace, 2005; Fixsen, Blase, Naoom, & Wallace, 2009). We discuss this parallel science-based development in Chaps. 8–11.

In these early debates, differences were sometimes unfortunately voiced or understood as if there was a binary choice to be made between delivery of *a process of evidence-based practice* and delivery of a *specific evidence-based treatment model*. Proponents of a process of evidence-based practice drew support from those who believed that eclectic approaches guided by practitioner creativity and experience were the best means to address the complexity of client situations (e.g., Green, 2008; Lucock et al., 2003). Critics of that belief noted the lack of evidence that eclectic practice was effective, as well as the challenges to implementing and sustaining it (Thyer, 2013).

For example, our eclectic school social worker in Chap. 2 had no organizational supports to know if he delivered Motivational Interviewing with fidelity. All he knew was that Tameisha's behaviors of concern were not improving. Therefore, he changed interventions to use a psychodynamic counseling approach, and then a behavioral approach, all without success. But what if Motivational Interviewing had been the correct selection of a proven intervention for that client and situation, but it wasn't delivered long enough or frequently enough, let alone with fidelity?

Ethically, eclectic practitioners should approach such questions carefully, using session data to inform consistent coaching or supervision to address these questions and determine best next steps. Our well-intentioned eclectic school social worker did not have such support. To refine knowledge and skills, he relied upon participation in continuing education workshops required for licensure. However, quality control mechanisms to monitor the content and delivery of continuing education workshops are relatively lax (Thyer & Pignotti, 2016).

Finally, consider this. Even when organizations hire experienced, effective eclectic practitioners, these practitioners change jobs or leave to marry or raise children. Eclectic approaches have many built-in constraints and challenges that are often not addressed. Furthermore, their proponents added opinions and beliefs to debates about evidence-based practice that reflected or amplified many misperceptions that we will address with facts in Chap. 4.

As these debates unfolded, purveyors (model developers) continued to clarify and prove first the efficacy, and then the effectiveness of specific practice models. Much like the emergence of family therapy in the 1960s and 1970s, treatment models emerged to address specific behavioral concerns that were not responding to more traditional counseling or case management approaches.

However, by the 1990s, the development of behavioral health care interventions and models followed a more disciplined scientific method of clearly identifying the population of concern, then clarifying elements and activities and phases of service delivery that included a theory of change, then demonstrating in small trials the efficacy of that model while also identifying means to evaluate fidelity of its delivery. With this foundation, the model could then be tested in random assignment experimental studies to establish its effectiveness.

Clear Definitions from Medicine

To understand differences, we must understand their context. Knowledge of history is critical to appreciate the context of any debate. Initial definitions of evidence-based practice (EBP) emerged from the field of medicine in the 1990s. Described as an explicit, judicious use of the best available scientific evidence to make decisions about patient care, evidence-based practice is well understood and accepted in medical education and services (Sackett, Rosenberg, Gray, Haynes, & Richardson, 1996; Straus, Glasziou, Richardson, & Haynes, 2011).

The Institute of Medicine (2001) summarized *the process of evidence-based practice* as the integration of best research evidence with clinical expertise *and* patient values (Institute of Medicine, 2001). Sackett (1997) delineated five steps that comprise *a process of evidence-based practice*:

1. **Convert the need for information into an answerable question.** For example; What might contribute to loss of appetite and listlessness in a previously active, gregarious African-American girl whose academic performance was diminishing and whose school behaviors were becoming disruptive?

2. **Find the best available evidence to answer that question**. In our child and family tale, the doctor examined Cochrane systematic reviews (www.cochrane.org), and ran a series of recommended tests that based on her expertise seemed warranted. She discovered a parasite and recommended a specific diet change concurrent with the medication most likely to eliminate the parasite.

3. **Critically evaluate the validity, impact, and applicability of that evidence to the client's circumstances**. This requires development of strong critical thinking abilities. In that child and family tale, the doctor discussed with the family how they had experienced significant disruptions in social support, in Tameisha's friendships, and related adjustments to new school and community contexts. The doctor cautioned that if the elimination of the parasite, and return of the girl's energy and appetite did not lead to improved academic performance and behavior, they should seek help at a behavioral healthcare clinic.

4. **Integrate relevant evidence with the practitioner's clinical expertise, client values and circumstances**. Although the doctor recommended a behavioral healthcare clinic, the family balked at the thought of seeking help in a mental health setting, so the doctor suggested they should work closely with school personnel.

5. **Evaluate how well the intervention was implemented, the outcomes achieved, and what should next occur**. The prescribed diet change combined with the medication improved the girl's appetite and energy. Since academic performance and school behaviors did not improve, the doctor recommended treatment at a behavioral healthcare clinic. When this did not fit with family concerns and values, the doctor recommended they work with school personnel.

> *We take such medical expertise in assessment and treatment for granted. We expect it. Effective doctors engage us in a collaborative assessment of contributing factors to our concerns. Applying a practical clinical wisdom born of years of experience, they discuss our concerns and identify proven means to address them.*

Process or Treatment Model?

In behavioral health care, Chambless and Ollendick (2001) as well as Silverman and Hinshaw (2008), defined *evidence-based practice models* as having:

(a) a clearly defined target population;

(b) specific written elements, activities, and phases of service delivery that,

(c) through random-assignment control group studies, demonstrates the effectiveness of that practice with that population.

Logically, this definition of *evidence-based practice models* seems intrinsically supportive and capable of being fully integrated within steps two and three of the definition of *a process of evidence-based practice*. Based upon client situation and characteristics, the practitioner should search for interventions or treatment models that are proven effective, then carefully examine their elements, activities, and phases of service delivery. In step four of *a process of evidence-based practice*, the clinician evaluates their ability to conduct these elements and activities in their organization, and discusses the treatment options with the client to ascertain best fit with client values and preferences.

Context and Concerns Across Disciplines

In the 1990s and through the turn of the century, process and model definitions of evidence-based practice emerged and were integrated into the science-driven field of medicine. However, disciplines addressing human behavior, especially those whose history was less defined by the scientific method, debated concepts, and definitions. Let us take a moment to briefly examine the historical context and concerns expressed in those disciplines' debates about definitions of evidence-based practice.

Social Work. Early twenty-first-century social work debates about evidence-based practice culminated in an edition of *The Journal of Research on Social Work Practice* devoted to papers and recommendations from a symposium of over 200 social work educators from 70 universities in the USA, Canada, and Sweden (Rubin, 2007). The event was inspired by findings from a survey of over 900 faculty from US MSW programs. Most respondents (73%) viewed evidence-based practice favorably, but identified significant definitional disparities and concerns about integrating evidence-based practice into the curriculum. Common concerns reflected faculty misconceptions such as:

- Evidence-based practices undervalue clinical expertise
- Client values and preferences may be ignored
- Evidence-based practice is not individualized for each client
- Evidence-based practices are used only for cost efficiency

Also noted was the lack of attention in social work research and discourse to the influence of organizational resources, policies, workload assignments, and components like training and supervision that can compromise delivery of empirically supported interventions and treatment models (Rubin, 2007; Rubin & Parrish, 2007). Some believed that evidence-based practices were not sufficiently tested with more complex client populations facing multiple issues, or that they failed to consider macro-socioeconomic factors like racism and poverty and thus might not be efficacious for the unique needs of diverse groups.

Early debates also noted that in some research designs, subjects might be dropped from analysis if there was co-morbidity of problems, and that these client populations are often the ones served by social workers (Otto, Polutta, & Ziegler, 2009). Others asserted that treatment manual specification of elements, activities, and phases of a service model, as well as measurements of fidelity, constrain clinician creativity (Addis, Wade, & Hatgis, 1999; Gitterman & Knight, 2013). Those expressing this perspective frequently noted that in studies of psychotherapy, the relationship between the client and clinician was identified as more efficacious than specific treatment interventions (Wampold, 2001; Wampold & Bhati, 2004).

In contrast, those advocating evidence-based practice asserted that thoughtful selection of interventions with clients and evaluation of intervention outcomes encouraged clients to be informed consumers, supported professional accountability to clients, and supported continual development of social work competencies (Gambrill, 1999, 2007; Hudson, 2009; Zlotnik, 2007). Parrish and Rubin (2012) suggested that as a discipline, social workers' attitudes about evidence-based practice were similar to other disciplines. These social work perspectives mirror more recent emphasis in medical literature that the best research evidence should be integrated with clinical expertise and with the patient's unique preferences, concerns, expectations, and circumstances (Straus, Glasziou, Richardson, & Haynes, 2011). Nevertheless, after more than a decade of clarification and debate, Gitterman and Knight (2013) remained critical of definitions of evidence-based practice in social work and of their origins in the field of medicine. However, Thyer's response (2013) addressed this rather dated critique by noting that the alternative was continued delivery of unproven practices.

The first article introducing the topic of evidence-based practice to a social work audience appeared in Families in Society: The Journal of Contemporary Social Services (Gambrill, 1999). Throughout the first decade of the twenty-first century, Gambrill clarified and presented ethical rationale for evidence-based practice in social work (Gambrill, 2007, 2010; Gambrill & Gibbs, 2009). Her contributions continue to this day (Gambrill, 2018).

Psychology, Marriage and Family Therapy. The discourse in social work paralleled that occurring in related professions. The American Psychological Association appointed a task force on evidence-based practice that asserted the purpose of evidence-based practice in psychology was to promote effective practice and to enhance public health by applying empirically supported principles of assessment, case formulation, therapeutic relationship, and intervention (2006). It defined evidence-based practice in psychology as the integration of the best available research with clinical expertise in the context of patient characteristics, culture, and preferences. Astute readers will note how this closely reflects the definition adopted by the Institute of Medicine (2001) from Sackett et al. (1996).

Marriage and family therapy education and training emerged from the development of systemic theories of behavior that challenged psychodynamic, individually focused practices. Psychodynamic theory itself emerged from Freud's scientifically unproven theory that was presented through anecdote and subjective reports of patient treatment. When family therapy pioneers articulated alternative models based in family systems theory (e.g., Bowen, 1978; Haley, 1987; Minuchin, Montalvo, Guerney, Rosman, & Schumer, 1967; Minuchin, 1974; Minuchin & Fishman, 1981), their presentations of new theory and practices also tended to be anecdotal or in case study format rather than examined and presented through random assignment controlled studies (Crane, Wampler, Sprenkle, Sandberg, & Hovestadt, 2002). This early model development progressed through the formation of family institutes that applied an apprenticeship approach to teaching new theories and techniques to student clinicians (Kaslow et al., 2007).

In 1995, a special issue of the *Journal of Marital and Family Therapy* (Pinsof & Wynne, 1995) provided an extensive review of the efficacy research on family therapy to date. The editors concluded that couple and family therapy is more effective than treatment that does not involve the family for a variety of behavioral and relational issues. However, there was insufficient data in meta-analytic studies to suggest the superiority of any particular form of family therapy (Shadish, Ragsdale, & Glaser, 1995).

As the field of behavioral health care focused on improving outcomes by addressing gaps between research and practice (Hoge et al., 2005), the American Association of Marriage and Family Therapists also created a task force to identify core competencies that should be developed through a process of evidence-informed, outcome-based education (Nelson et al., 2007).

> *Thus, through the first decade of the twenty-first century, social work, psychology, marriage and family therapy and the field of behavioral health care were focused on improving outcomes, addressing the gap between research and practice, and on clarifying definitions of evidence-based practice.*

A Process of Evidence-Based Practice

In that historical period, Rubin (2007) provided a very simple description of evidence-based practice as a social worker's selection and use of practice methods that have clear evidence to support improving outcomes in a specific client population. Astute readers will note parallels with the definition offered by Chambless and Ollendick (2001) for defining an *evidence-based treatment model*.

Nevertheless, several authors suggested very similar steps to inculcate the medical definition of *the process of evidence-based practice* in social work values and ethics (Gibbs & Gambrill, 2002; Thyer & Pignotti, 2011). The steps are remarkably comparable to those asserted by Sackett et al. (1997) and the Institute of Medicine (2001). They include:

1. **Identification of an answerable question**

For example: What might contribute to a previously pro-social, well-engaged African-American female student's diminished academic performance and disruptive school behaviors?

2. **Find evidence to address that question**

This requires development of knowledge and skills for searching secondary source registries such as Blueprints for Healthy Youth Development, or the California Clearinghouse for Evidence-Based Practice in Child Welfare, or the Campbell Collaboration, as well as searching peer-reviewed, evidence-informed literature.

3. **Critical review of the scientific validity and strength of that evidence**

This ability should be well developed in the academic curricula of social work and related disciplines.

4. **Use of clinical expertise to compare that evidence with client values before choosing to apply it in practice**

In our Chap. 2 example, this occurred with the MST practitioner but did not with the school social worker.

5. **Subsequent evaluation with clients of the effectiveness of the intervention and its outcomes**

In our Chap. 2 example, outcome evaluation with clients occurred in delivery of MST, but not in the school-initiated interventions.

Evidence-Based Practice Models

Concurrent with early academic debates about *a process of evidence-based practice*, there were also debates about definitions for *evidence-based treatment models*. These debates coalesced around the amount or type of evidence necessary, the clarity and thoroughness of descriptions for the treatment model, and the specificity about populations for which it was proven effective.

We have previously presented the classic definition of an evidence-based practice model. It must have: (a) clearly defined target population; (b) a written description of the participants, elements, activities, and phases of service delivery; and (c) research supporting effectiveness with that population established through random-assignment control group studies (Chambless & Ollendick, 2001; Silverman & Hinshaw, 2008).

This definition requires time and resources to refine and describe the participants, elements, activities, and phases of service delivery, and if delivered with fidelity, how change occurs (theory of change). Through an example in Chap. 6, we present how model development and testing with measures of fidelity requires efficacy studies before it is ready for random assignment control group studies. Efficacy trials help to refine the practice model, to establish means for evaluating fidelity in its delivery, while also measuring outcomes. Random assignment control group studies maintain fidelity in the better-defined model and address the process supporting its implementation while comparing its outcomes to those produced from other practices with the same client population.

Critics and skeptics asserted that in the time it takes to refine a practice, establish its efficacy, and then test its effectiveness with a specific population, too many clients might receive less than efficacious practices when current interventions may be sufficient (Huey & Polo, 2008). However, as more and more practice models for a variety of behavioral concerns establish a rigorous evidence base, and as frameworks to apply them in diverse contexts emerge (e.g., Bernal, Jiménez-Chafey, & Domenech Rodríguez, 2009; Lau, 2006), this perspective is losing valence.

Other critics and skeptics noted that developers of some evidence-based practices required proprietary processes to ensure implementation quality. Many asserted this could be too expensive. All too often these assertions were made without examining efficiency (more clients achieving improved and sustainable outcomes) or without examining longitudinal cost-benefit analysis (Dopp, Borduin, Wagner, & Sawyer, 2014). Or, as Thyer (2013) noted in pointed response to Gitterman's and Knight's criticisms of evidence-based practice in social work, the alternative is to deliver business-as-usual which has no proven effectiveness.

These concerns and critiques were not solely academic debates within disciplines. Some practice models with limited studies of effectiveness also asserted new terminology. For example, for some time proponents of Wraparound asserted it was a "practice-based evidence" model (Walker & Bruns, 2006).

To differentiate specific evidence-based practice models with more limited research, several authors proposed terms such as "evidence supported treatment," "promising practice," and "evidence-informed interventions." (Gibbs & Gambrill, 2002; Thyer & Myers, 2011; Thyer & Pignotti, 2011).

Many of these confusing definitional terms were well-meant attempts to address the time it takes to establish evidence of effectiveness. They were also products of the lack of common criteria for the amount or types of evidence necessary to warrant use of the term "evidence-based practice."

Definitions by Extent of Evidence

Science advances more slowly amidst confusing and changing definitions and terms. We have presented how descriptions of elements and activities in specific steps in *a process of evidence-based practice* were relatively aligned across disciplines. Although one of these steps required the practitioner to critically examine the scientific validity and strength of that evidence, specific criteria were not asserted. We have also presented how the definitions and terms used to describe *evidence-based practice or treatment models* at first lacked criteria for the extent of studies necessary to differentiate its validity and strength.

The highly regarded Blueprints for Healthy Youth Development presents a "continuum of confidence in evidence of effectiveness" that can help faculty, students, practitioners, and program administrators differentiate the extent to which an intervention or a practice model is evidence-based (https://www.blueprintsprograms.com/standards-of-evidence). The Blueprints continuum of confidence in evidence of effectiveness includes:

Opinion informed. Evidence with the lowest level of confidence is opinion informed. This includes anecdotal or testimonial information from a few individuals. Though usually based on a larger sample, satisfaction surveys also seek opinions of a program. Such evidence may be somewhat useful in early stages of program development, but there is no systematic evaluation of outcomes.

Research informed. Research-informed studies gather outcome data from surveys or agency records, or even records from other systems (e.g., school attendance, behavior, and academic performance). If a survey is administered at program entry and exit, this provides some evidence of effectiveness, but the level of confidence remains low because surveys or agency records cannot isolate the intervention's impact from other possible influences on intended outcomes. Also, with no control or comparison group, outcomes cannot be attributed to the program.

Correlational studies can reveal if a positive relationship, a negative relationship, or no relationship exists between a program and a desired outcome. However, demonstrating that a relationship exists does not identify or demonstrate which elements or activities contributed to outcomes.

Correlation is not causation. There is always the possibility that unexamined additional factors influenced correlation between an examined factor and the outcome. For example, if researchers find a positive correlation between self-efficacy and treatment outcomes, they would not know if the intervention improved self-efficacy and therefore influenced treatment outcomes. It could also be that regardless of treatment elements and activities, baseline levels of self-efficacy were already sufficient. It could also be that regardless of treatment elements and activities, those completing treatment felt greater self-efficacy just for finishing. Correlational studies can be useful to ensure that treatments are not causing harm, or that there is an association between the treatment and those factors hypothesized to make a difference in treatment effects, but correlational studies alone are not sufficient to label an intervention "evidence-based."

Evidence-based programs. For programs or practices that warrant the term "evidence-based," there are differing degrees of confidence in the evidence. For example, quasi-experimental designs do not use random assignment and therefore lack certainty that the treatment and control groups are equivalent at the start of the study. Comparison groups may be matched on measured characteristics but still may differ on characteristics that were not considered or measured. Thus, a potential for bias remains, and confidence in the evidence of effectiveness remains moderate.

Virtually all web-based registries of evidence-based practices (see to the Appendix of Registries) place the greatest confidence in evidence derived from experimental study designs because they include control groups that do not receive the program intervention. If participants receiving the program intervention have better outcomes than those in the control group, then the program is likely the cause of this desired effect. Levels of confidence and evidence of effectiveness from experimental studies may vary from moderate to very high.

The highest level of confidence in evidence of effectiveness comes from multiple studies that demonstrate improved outcomes in different settings of randomly assigned subjects. Consistent findings across different sites greatly reduce the possibility that chance explains differences between intervention and control groups. This increases confidence to scale up the practice model across an entire organization or service system. Confidence increases further when investigators independent of the program developer, with no financial interests, conduct the studies.

Differentiating Program Models Based on Evidence

Blueprints program criteria. The Blueprints for Healthy Youth Development website also provides a registry of evidence-based programs that promote behavioral health and well-being of children and adolescents. These programs are family, school, and community-based. It includes a continuum of practice models, from primary prevention programs to secondary or tertiary prevention programs for at-risk children and youth. Applying the Blueprints continuum of confidence criteria, evidence-based programs are organized into only two categories, Promising Programs and Model Programs (https://www.blueprintsprograms.com).

Promising Programs meet the following criteria:

Intervention specificity. A written program description clearly identifies the targeted population and the outcome it is designed to achieve, as well as the targeted risk and/or protective factors, and how intervention components produce this outcome. This is also called a theory of change.
Evaluation quality. At least one high-quality randomized control trial or two high-quality quasi-experimental evaluations produce valid and reliable findings.
Intervention impact. The preponderance of evidence indicates significant improvement in intended outcomes that can be attributed to the program and there is no evidence of harmful effects.
Dissemination readiness. The program or practice model identifies the necessary organizational capability. It provides manuals, training, technical assistance, and other support required for implementation with fidelity in communities and service systems.

Model Programs meet the above criteria and these additional standards:

Evaluation quality and sustainability. At least two high-quality randomized control trials or one high-quality randomized control trial plus one high-quality quasi-experimental evaluation demonstrate improved intended outcomes that are sustained for a minimum of 12 months.

Independent replication. In at least one of these studies, authorship, data collection and analysis were conducted by an evaluator who is neither a current or past member of the program developer's research team and who has no financial interest in the program.

Washington State Institute of Public Policy. To address the proliferation of confusing definitions and terms while simultaneously acknowledging concerns about criteria, the Washington State Institute for Public Policy (WSIPP) and the University of Washington Evidence-Based Practices Institute (EBPI) suggested three types of evidence-informed practices. This is the only registry that specifically requires programs that meet the highest evidence standards to have sufficient evaluations that include diverse research samples.

Evidence-based practice. They identify an evidence-based psychosocial intervention (EBP) as having four primary elements (WSIPP & EBPI, 2012):

1. Multiple randomized or statistically controlled evaluations, or one large multiple-site randomized or statistically controlled evaluation that demonstrates sustained improvements;
2. Practices engage an ethnically heterogeneous sample (at least 32% non-white);
3. Practice steps are clearly articulated for easy replication; and
4. Cost-benefit is reported.

The WSIPP definition is more expansive than the classic definition articulated by Chambless and Ollendick (2001) or Silverman and Hinshaw (2008) and includes factors that may inform policy decisions. It emphasizes systematic research but does not require multiple randomized controlled trials or follow-up assessment as do other secondary source repositories.

This definition includes considerations of concern to administrators, policy-makers and the public, specifically cost savings and the heterogeneity of population studied. For example, some proven practices may be more expensive than the cost savings from anticipated clinical, educational, or system-level outcomes (e.g., Families and Schools Together; WSIPP & EBPI, 2014). It also addresses concerns raised that some studies do not examine outcomes in populations of color (Sue, Zane, Nagayama Hall, & Berger, 2009). In fact, ensuring representative inclusion in research studies is now part of the National Institutes of Health (NIH) reporting requirements.

Research-based practice. Often developed in smaller programs outside of university settings, newer practice models will take time meet this definition of evidence-based practice. When there is less rigorous research but there are indications a practice model has, or is likely to have, favorable results, it may fit the category of a research-based practice (WSIPP/EBPI, 2012). A research-based practice may have one randomized or statistically controlled evaluation, or there may have been adequate random controlled studies, but due to lack of client heterogeneity, or to lack of testing and demonstrating cost-benefit, the practice model does not meet the more demanding criteria for an evidence-based model.

Promising practice. Finally, there are emerging practice models that through a case study or through reported but not systematically examined outcomes shows promise. A promising practice shows potential for efficacy and for meeting more demanding criteria, but simply has not yet been adequately studied.

The California Evidence-Based Clearinghouse for Child Welfare. The Chadwick Center for Children & Families at Rady Children's Hospital in San Diego houses this repository of information to support effective selection and implementation of evidence-based practices. Although funded by California, its focus is not limited to that state. More than 23,000 people from the USA and more than 190 countries visit the site each month (Nwabuzor Ogbonnaya, Martin, & Walsh, 2018). Practice models are systematically examined and rated using the following criteria:

Well supported by research evidence (1). At least two rigorous random controlled trials (RCT) in different settings found the practice model to be superior (improved outcomes) to an appropriate comparison practice. When compared to a control group in at least one of the studies, improved outcomes were sustained for at least one year after the end of treatment.

Supported by research evidence (2). At least one rigorous RCT found the practice model to be superior (improved outcomes) to an appropriate comparison practice, and sustained those outcomes for at least six months beyond the end of treatment.

Promising research evidence (3). This rating is more complex. At least one study using some form of control (e.g., untreated group, placebo group, matched wait list) established improved outcomes over the control group. Additionally, its outcomes are comparable or superior to other practice models rated at this level or higher, or its outcomes are superior to an appropriate comparison practice.

Evidence fails to demonstrate effect (4). When compared to usual care, two or more randomized, controlled outcome studies found that the practice model did not improve outcomes. If multiple outcome studies have been conducted, the overall weight of evidence does not support the benefit of the practice.

Concerning practice (5). There is a legal or empirical basis suggesting that compared to its likely benefits, the practice constitutes a risk of harm to those receiving it. If multiple outcome studies have been conducted, the overall weight of evidence suggests the practice has a negative effect on clients. Case data suggest a risk of harm that was probably caused by the treatment and the harm was severe or frequent.

NR: not able to be rated. The practice does not have any published, peer-reviewed study using some form of control (e.g., untreated group, placebo group, matched wait list) that has established the practice's benefit over the placebo or found it to be comparable to or better than an appropriate comparison practice.

Family First Prevention Services Act of 2018

As we are writing this book, the importance of definitions and criteria for evidence-based practices is emerging on a national scale. To highlight how criteria and terms are increasingly more similar than different, as well as how major funding sources increasingly expect delivery of proven practices, we provide a brief description of the Family First Prevention Services Act (FFPSA) that was signed into law as part of the Bipartisan Budget Act (H.R. 1892) on February 9, 2018. FFPSA enables States to use Federal funds available under parts B and E of title IV of the Social Security Act to provide enhanced support to children and families and to prevent foster care placements through the provision of evidence-based mental health and substance abuse prevention and treatment services, in-home parent skill-based programs, and kinship navigator services.

By requiring the use of proven practices, this Act will have significant influence in both public and private child welfare service delivery. All practices must have a book, manual, or other written descriptions of the practice protocol components as well as how to administer the practice. It prioritizes programs or services that have implementation training and staff support and/or fidelity monitoring tools and resources. In section 471(e)(4)(C) FFPSA designates services as "promising," "supported," or "well-supported" practices as follows:

Promising practice. A promising practice is superior to an appropriate comparison practice. Superiority is demonstrated by at least one study using conventional standards of statistical significance in validated measures of important child and parent outcomes, such as mental health, substance abuse, and child safety and well-being. The study must use some form of control such as an untreated group, a placebo group, or a wait-list study.

Supported practice. A supported practice is established by at least one study that was rated well-designed and well-executed by an independent systematic review, as a rigorous random-controlled trial, or, a rigorous quasi-experimental research design. The study must be conducted in a usual care setting, and must establish that the practice has a sustained effect for at least six months beyond the end of treatment.

Well-supported practice. A well-supported practice is established by at least two studies, one of which demonstrates a sustained effect for at least one year beyond the end of treatment. It's important to note that the studies still need to be in usual care settings and evaluated by the independent systematic review.

Common Factors or Elements

Progress toward integrating evidence-based practice in professional degree programs was slow amidst the initial confusing plethora of definitions, terms, opinions, and beliefs. In Chap. 5, we present studies that discuss contributing factors to slow curricula transformation. However, one very practical concern voiced by hesitant faculty was the large number of courses required by accrediting bodies (Bertram, Charnin, Kerns, & Long, 2015). Those voicing this perspective approached teaching evidence-based practice as additive rather than integrative to existing curricula.

To address this concern and bridge the growing and confusing stream of definitions and terms, Barth et al. (2012) proposed that academic programs should teach a common factors or common elements approach. They asserted that protocols for evidence-based practice models share common phases, elements, and activities. Thus, instead of selecting certain practice models for inclusion in academic curricula, their common phases, elements, and activities could instead be integrated into courses.

While this seemed exceptionally logical, there were differing emphases and potential conflicting perspectives. The *common elements framework* (Chorpita, Daleiden, & Weisz, 2005; Chorpita, Becker, & Daleiden, 2007) conceptualized clinical practice as having common components and procedures drawn from many distinct practice model treatment protocols. The *common factors framework* (Duncan, Miller, Wampold, & Hubble, 2010; Sparks & Muro, 2009) asserted that the therapeutic alliance, client motivation, and practitioner factors common to all therapeutic interventions are responsible for treatment outcomes to a greater extent than are the elements and activities described in protocols for evidence-based practice models.

Astute readers will note that our school social worker in Chap. 2 participated in continuing education workshops that emphasized the therapeutic alliance as *the* driver of change. We will discuss this common assertion when we address misconceptions about evidence-based practice in Chap. 4. We will also discuss the implementation challenges and limitations of a common factors or common elements approach in later chapters.

Overlooked Questions

We previously noted that these early definitional debates treated the social worker or clinician as though they practiced independently. Many applicants to MSW programs or related disciplines desire to have their own private practice. However, most graduates are employed by organizations. Increasingly, funding sources require these organizations to deliver services proven to produce meaningful, improved client outcomes. To receive funding, these organizations must clearly describe the nature of their interventions with clients and how this improves client outcomes. Since the emergence of implementation science and frameworks (Fixsen et al., 2005; Bertram, Blase, & Fixsen, 2015), funding sources increasingly require grant or contract proposals to describe a theory of change that includes how the organization selects, develops, and supports workforce to deliver an ***evidence-based practice*** effectively and with fidelity. We will discuss theory of change in Chap. 8.

Discussion of organization and funding contexts was often absent in early evidence-based practice debates. This omission left several questions unanswered. If an organization has adopted a specific evidence-based practice, can employees engage in *a process of evidence-based practice*? If working in a private practice, how does the clinician know that interventions they use are delivered effectively with fidelity? If the clinician works in an organization that allows use of a common elements approach or the use of *a process of evidence-based practice*, how does the organization know the selected interventions are delivered effectively with fidelity? In such a situation, how does the organization supervise and coach the use of so many interventions? These questions reflect concerns about implementation. In Chaps. 8–11, we present implementation science and frameworks that emerged concurrently with the early debates about evidence-based practice.

Summary

In the first decade of the twenty-first century, amidst debates about evidence-based practice, there was an increasing emphasis on achieving improved client and public health outcomes by addressing the gap between research and practice. However, there was debate about definitions and criteria for evidence-based practice. Did that term describe a process of practice or specific treatment models? Gradually consensus emerged that the answer to both questions was "yes" and that whether a process or a specific treatment model could be selected for delivery was very much dependent upon organizational and contextual factors.

In the second decade of the twenty-first century, consensus is emerging about terms and criteria for the extent of evidence necessary to differentiate less-proven from well-proven practices. The Blueprints' continuum of confidence in evidence provides very helpful guidance. It is logical, easily taught and understood. It provides a science-based rationale for each term that parallels the emerging consensus of terms and definitions applied by the Washington State Institute for Public Policy (WSIPP) and the University of Washington Evidence-Based Practices Institute (EBPI), by Blueprints themselves, and by the California Evidence-Based Clearinghouse for child welfare. This emerging consensus is reflected in the recently passed Family First Prevention Services Act.

Nevertheless, myth and misconceptions about evidence-based practice continue to be expressed by many faculty in professional degree programs as well as by many staff in behavioral healthcare or social service programs and systems. In the next chapter, we briefly address these myths and misconceptions with facts. Then, in Chap. 5, we examine workforce preparation by professional degree programs.

References

Addis, M., Wade, W. A., & Hatgis, C. (1999). Barriers to dissemination of evidence-based practices: Addressing practitioners' concerns about manual-based psychotherapies. *Clinical Psychology: Science and Practice, 6,* 430–441.

American Psychological Association Presidential Task Force on Evidence Based-Practice. (2006). Evidence-based practice in psychology. *American Psychologist, 61*(4), 271–285. https://doi.org/10.1037/0003-066x.61.4.271.

Barth, R. P., Lee, B. R., Lindsey, M. A., Collins, K. S., Strieder, F., Chorpita, B. F., et al. (2012). Evidence-based practice at a crossroads: The timely emergence of common elements and common factors. *Research on Social Work Practice, 22*(1), 108–119.

Bernal, G., Jiméncz-Chafey, M. I., & Domenech Rodríguez, M. M. (2009). Cultural adaptation of treatments: A resource for considering culture in evidence-based practice. *Professional Psychology: Research and Practice, 40*(4), 361.

Bertram, R. M., Blase, K. A., & Fixsen, D. L. (2015a). Improving programs and outcomes: Implementation frameworks and organization change. *Research on Social Work Practice, 25*(4), 477–487.

Bertram, R. M., Charnin, L. A., Kerns, S. E. U., & Long, A. C. (2015b). Evidence-based practices in North American MSW curricula. *Research on Social Work Practice, 25*(6), 737–748.

Bowen, M. (1978). *Family Therapy in Clinical Practice*. NY and London: Jason Aronson.

Chambless, D. L., & Ollendick, T. H. (2001). Empirically supported psychological interventions: Controversies and evidence. *Annual Review of Psychology, 52*, 685–716.

Chorpita, B. F., Becker, K. D., & Daleiden, E. L. (2007). Understanding the common elements of evidence based practice: Misconceptions and clinical examples. *Journal of the American Academy of Child and Adolescent Psychiatry, 46*, 647–652.

Chorpita, B. F., Daleiden, E., & Weisz, J. R. (2005). Identifying and selecting the common elements of evidence based interventions: A distillation and matching model. *Mental Health Services Research, 7*, 5–20.

Crane, D. R., Wampler, K. S., Sprenkle, D. H., Sandberg, J. G., & Hovestadt, A. J. (2002). The scientist-practitioner model in marriage and family therapy doctoral programs. *Journal of Marital and Family Therapy, 28*, 75–83.

Dopp, A. R., Borduin, C. M., Wagner, D. V., & Sawyer, A. M. (2014). The economic impact of multisystemic therapy through midlife: A cost–benefit analysis with serious juvenile offenders and their siblings. *Journal of Consulting and Clinical Psychology, 82*(4), 694.

Duncan, B. L., Miller, S. D., Wampold, B. E., & Hubble, M. A. (2010). *The heart and soul of change: Delivering what works* (2nd ed.). Washington, DC: American Psychological Association.

Fixsen, D. L., Blase, K. A., Naoom, S. F., & Wallace, F. (2009). Core implementation components. *Research on Social Work Practice, 19*(5), 531–540.

Fixsen, D. L., Naoom, S. F., Blase, K. A., Friedman, R. M., & Wallace, F. (2005). *Implementation research: A synthesis of the literature*. Tampa, FL: University of South Florida, Louis de la Parte Florida Mental Health Institute, The National Implementation Research Network (FMHI Publication #231).

Gambrill, E. (1999). Evidence-based practice: An alternative to authority-based practice. *Families in Society: The Journal of Contemporary Human Services, 80*, 341–350. https://doi.org/10.1606/1044-3894.1214.

Gambrill, E. (2007). Views of evidence-based practice: Social workers' code of ethics and accreditation standards as guides for choice. *Journal of Social Work Education, 43*, 447–462.

Gambrill, E., & Gibbs, L. (2009). Developing well-structured questions for evidence-informed practice. In A. R. Roberts (Ed.), *Social workers' desk reference* (2nd ed., pp. 1120–1126). New York, NY: Oxford University Press.

Gambrill, E. (2010). Evidence-informed practice: Antidote to propaganda in the helping profession. *Research on Social Work Practice, 20*, 302–320.

Gambrill, E. (2018). Contributions of the process of evidence-based practice to implementation: Educational opportunities. *Journal of Social Work Education, 54*(sup1), S113–S125.

Gibbs, L., & Gambrill, E. (2002). Evidence-based practice: Counterarguments to objections. *Research on Social Work Practice, 12*(3), 452–476.

Gitterman, A., & Knight, C. (2013). Evidence-guided practice: Integrating the science and art of social work. *Families in Society: The Journal of Contemporary Social Services, 94*, 70–78.

Green, L. W. (2008). Making research relevant: If it is an evidence-based practice, where's the practice-based evidence?. *Family Practice, 25*(suppl_1), i20–i24.

Haley, J. (1987). *The Jossey-Bass social and behavioral science series. Problem-solving therapy* (2nd ed.). San Francisco, CA, US: Jossey-Bass.

Hoge, M. A., Morris, J. A., Daniels, A. S., Huey, L. Y., Stuart, G. W., Adams, N., et al. (2005). Report of recommendations: The Annapolis coalition conference on behavioral health work force competencies. *Administration and Policy in Mental Health and Mental Health Services Research, 32*(5–6), 651–663.

Hudson, C. (2009). Decision-making in evidence-based practice: Science and art. *Smith College Studies in Social Work, 79,* 155–174.

Huey, S. J., Jr., & Polo, A. J. (2008). Evidence-based psychosocial treatments for ethnic minority youth. *Journal of Clinical Child & Adolescent Psychology, 37*(1), 262–301.

Institute of Medicine. (2001). *Crossing the quality chasm: A new healthy system for the 21st Century.* Washington, DC: National Academic Press.

Kaslow, N. J., Rubin, N. J., Forrest, L., Elman, N. S., Van Horne, B. A., Jacobs, S. C., et al. (2007). Recognizing, assessing, and intervening with problems of professional competence. *Professional Psychology: Research and Practice, 38*(5), 479–492.

Lau, A. S. (2006). Making the case for selective and directed cultural adaptations of evidence-based treatments: Examples from parent training. *Clinical Psychology: Science and Practice, 13*(4), 295–310.

Lucock, M., Leach, C., Iveson, S., Lynch, K., Horsefield, C., & Hall, P. (2003). A systematic approach to practice-based evidence in a psychological therapies service. *Clinical Psychology & Psychotherapy: An International Journal of Theory & Practice, 10*(6), 389–399.

Minuchin, S. (1974). *Families & Family Therapy*. Cambridge, MA: Harvard University Press.

Minuchin, S., Montalvo, B., Guerney, B., Rosman, B., & Schumer, F. (1967). *Families of the slums*. New York: Basic Books.

Minuchin, S., & Fishman, H. C. (1981). *Family therapy techniques*. Cambridge, MA: Harvard University Press.

Nelson, T. S., Chenail, R. J., Alexander, J. F., Crane, D. R., Johnson, S. M., & Schwallie, L. (2007). The development of core competencies for the practice of marriage and family therapy. *Journal of Marital and Family Therapy, 33*(4), 417–438.

Nwabuzor Ogbonnaya, I., Martin, J., & Walsh, C. R. (2018). Using the California Evidence-based clearinghouse for child welfare as a tool for teaching evidence-based practice. *Journal of Social Work Education, 54*(sup1), S31–S40.

Otto, H. U., Polutta, A., & Ziegler, H. (2009). Reflexive professionalism as a second generation of evidence-based practice: Some considerations on the special issue "What works? Modernizing the knowledge-base of social work". *Research on Social Work Practice, 19,* 472–478.

Parrish, D. E., & Rubin, A. (2012). Social workers' orientations toward the evidence-based practice process: A comparison with psychologists and licensed marriage and family therapists. *Social Work, 57*(3), 201–210.

Pinsof, W., & Wynne, L. (Eds.). (1995). Special issue: The effectiveness of marital and family therapy. *Journal of Marital and Family Therapy, 21*(4).

Rubin, A. (2007). Improving the teaching of evidence-based practice: Introduction to the special issue. *Research on Social Work Practice, 17*(5), 541–547.

Rubin, A., & Parrish, D. (2007). Views of evidence-based practice among faculty in master of social work programs: A national survey. *Research on Social Work Practice, 17*(1), 110–122.

Sackett, D. L. (1997). February). *Evidence-based medicine. Seminars in Perinatology, 21*(1), 3–5.

Sackett, D. L., Rosenberg, W. M., Gray, J. M., Haynes, R. B., & Richardson, W. S. (1996). Evidence based medicine: What it is and what it isn't. *Clinical Orthopaedics and Related Research, 455,* 3–5.

Shadish, W. R., Ragsdale, K., Glaser, R. R., & Montgomery, L. M. (1995). The efficacy and effectiveness of marital and family therapy: A perspective from meta-analysis. *Journal of Marital and Family Therapy, 21*(4), 345–360.

Silverman, W. K., & Hinshaw, S. P. (2008). The second special issue on evidence-based psychosocial treatments for children and adolescents: A 10-year update. *Journal of Clinical Child and Adolescent Psychology, 37,* 1–7.

Sparks, J. A., & Muro, M. L. (2009). Client-directed wraparound: The client as connector in community collaboration. *Journal of Systemic Therapies, 28,* 63–76.

Straus, S. E., Glasziou, P., Richardson, W. S., & Haynes, R. B. (2011). *Evidence-based medicine: How to practice and teach it* (4th ed.). New York, NY: Churchill Livingstone.

Sue, S., Zane, N., Nagayama Hall, G. C., & Berger, L. K. (2009). The case for cultural competency in psychotherapeutic interventions. *Annual Review of Psychology, 60,* 525–548.

Thyer, B. (2013). Evidence-based practice or evidence-guided practice: A rose by any other name would smell as sweet [Invited response to Gitterman & Knight's "Evidence-guided practice"]. *Families in Society: The Journal of Contemporary Social Services, 94*(2), 79–84.

Thyer, B. A., & Myers, L. L. (2011). The quest for evidence-based practice: A view from the United States. *Journal of Social Work, 11,* 8–25.

Thyer, B. A., & Pignotti, M. (2016). The problem of pseudoscience in social work continuing education. *Journal of Social Work Education, 52*(2), 136–146.

Walker, J. S., & Bruns, E. J. (2006). Building on practice-based evidence: Using expert perspectives to define the wraparound process. *Psychiatric Services, 57*(11), 1579–1585.

Wampold, B. (2001). *The great psychotherapy debate.* Mahwah, NJ: Lawrence Erlbaum.

Wampold, B. E., & Bhati, K. S. (2004). Attending to the omissions: A historical examination of evidence-based practice movements. *Professional Psychology: Research and Practice, 35,* 563–570.

Washington State Institute for Public Policy and University of Washington Evidence Based Practices Institute. (2012). *Inventory of evidence-based, research-based, and promising practices.* Report ID: E2SHB2536.

Zlotnik, J. (2007). Evidence-based practice and social work education: A view from Washington. *Research on Social Work Practice, 17,* 625–629.

Chapter 4
Misconceptions and Facts

Here, for a brief moment, we pause to paraphrase the opening paragraph of this book. The scientific method is being ignored or minimized when proven facts seem confusing or uncomfortable. Myths and misconceptions are passionately asserted to challenge science when findings suggest a new and necessary path that may disrupt accustomed practice and belief. In this through the looking glass historical moment, opinion, or faith are often asserted as alternatives to avert inconvenient truths. In this chapter, we present facts that address the myths and misconceptions that fuel inaccurate opinions and beliefs about evidence-based practice. These myths and misperceptions emerged in the early debates about evidence-based practice. While some have lost their valence, others continue to this day and shape the thinking of academic faculty and behavioral health care or social service program administrators, managers, supervisors, and practitioners.

The requirement that an *evidence-based treatment model* should have a written description of its participants, elements, and activities in phases of service delivery is a lodestone for many misconceptions that reflect and contribute to the plethora of terms and definitions for evidence-based practice. The requirement that a practice model be proven effective in random assignment controlled studies with a clearly defined target population also contributed to misconceptions that tempered enthusiasm and constrained the adoption of evidence-based practices in behavioral health care as well as their integration into academic and field curricula of professional degree programs. Common myths and related misconceptions coalesce around the following concerns.

Misconception: Restrictive Criteria

This misconception is a product of early debates about evidence-based practice. Opponents focused on the Chambless and Ollendick (2001) criteria that an evidence-based treatment model must clearly identify its target population have a written manual or guidelines and be proven effective in random-controlled studies. Critics

© Springer Nature Switzerland AG 2019
R. Bertram and S. Kerns, *Selecting and Implementing Evidence-Based Practice*,
https://doi.org/10.1007/978-3-030-11325-4_4

complained that this process takes time and resources that a service organization usually does not have to prove that its approach is effective.

> *Related to this definition, misconceptions emerged around the importance of the therapeutic relationship, as well as the importance of practitioner expertise and creativity. These myths and misconceptions are addressed separately in this chapter.*

Facts. In the previous chapter, we highlighted ways in which the field has matured and grown from early debates. While there is no universally adopted definition of evidence-based practice, there are now recognized gradations that describe a continuum of evidence supporting a treatment model. All practices can and are being organized in a continuum from "harmful" to "no evidence" from "limited research but promising," to "research-based," to "multiple randomized clinical trials." Criteria for differentiating these gradations of evidence supporting a treatment model are remarkably and increasingly similar. In the previous chapter, we reviewed these similarities of gradation as evidenced in the newly initiated Family First Prevention Services Act, in the criteria and terms developed by the Washington State Institute for Public Policy (WSIPP) and the University of Washington Evidence-Based Practices Institute (EBPI), in criteria and terms used by the California Evidence-Based Clearinghouse for Child Welfare, and in the Blueprints for Healthy Youth Development's continuum of confidence in evidence. This continuum of evidence supporting intervention practices should be clearly presented in professional degree programs that produce practitioners, supervisors, managers, and administrators for behavioral health care and social service programs and systems.

Misconception: Single Behavioral Concern

Another common myth that emerged from the criteria for evidence-based treatment models was the belief that these practice models are designed to only address a single behavioral health concern. This misconception stems in part from the requirement that a practice be proven effective for a well-defined target population. It may also reflect assumptions that randomized controlled trials do not accept clients with comorbid conditions or that they eliminate results if a client experiences comorbid conditions (e.g., if a model was designed to address disruptive youth behavior, but the study eliminated results for disruptive youth if they also used marijuana or alcohol) or that these studies only examine a single life domain (e.g., only evaluating school behavior and performance but not examining behavioral outcomes at home or in the community).

Facts. Most *evidence-supported treatment models* can address multiple behaviors of concern and achieve positive outcomes across multiple domains in a person's life, such as school/job attendance and performance, living at home, staying out of the justice system, improved behavioral self-regulation, and parent–child relationships. This is also true for *evidence-based practice models* addressing adult behavioral concerns. There is even some evidence that interventions addressing parenting behaviors can diminish parental depression (e.g., Nowak & Heinrichs, 2008). The Campbell Collaboration (http://www.campbellcollaboration.org) and the Cochrane Collaboration (http://www.cochrane.org) offer many examples of complex health and social problems that have been extensively investigated using high-quality research studies. Regular reviews of literature maintain and update these repositories of information.

Misconception: Client Diversity

While the concern that practices must be proven for diverse populations is quite appropriate and understandable, an often-asserted myth is the belief that evidence-based practices are not developed for diverse client populations. Like the single behavioral concern myth, this misconception stems from the requirement that a practice be proven effective for a well-defined target population. Like the single behavioral concern myth, it is also linked with the assumption that random assignment controlled studies eliminate results of clients with comorbid conditions, and people living in diverse and lower income communities must often address more than a single concern. Finally, the belief that evidence-based practices are not developed for diverse populations may be linked with assumptions that random assignment controlled studies are university-based rather than community-based.

Facts. There has been significant progress in understanding how evidence-based practices work for a variety of populations. Many *evidence-supported treatment models* achieve excellent results with a variety of population demographics and with more than a single problem focus. They emphasize careful assessment of unique factors shaping behaviors of concern and of youth, family, and ecological strengths that can promote and support change. Also, many evidence-based practices were developed for specific racial and ethnic groups and/or studied with diverse clientele. Huey and Polo (2008) identified evidence-supported treatments for ethnic minority youth, identifying those that address anxiety, depression, trauma, substance use, and conduct problems, as well as concurrent behavior and emotional problems. Furthermore, since the 1990s, Multisystemic Therapy (MST) has been tested in communities, adapted and successfully provided for different populations including psychiatric crisis (Henggeler et al., 1999), juvenile sex offenders (Letourneau et al., 2009), child abuse and neglect (Swenson, Schaeffer, Henggeler, Faldowski, & Mayhew, 2010), and youth transitioning from secure incarceration (Trupin, Kerns, Walker, DeRobertis, & Stewart, 2011).

Misconception: Client Values and Choice

Especially in the early debates, many asserted the belief that evidence-based practices ignore client values and limit or do not consider client preferences (choice). This misconception was shaped by the requirement that an *evidence-based treatment model* should specify the participants, elements, and activities in phases of service delivery. Strong objections to so-called manualized treatment were expressed by Straus and McAlister (2000) and Webb (2001). Some of those authors also asserted the inaccurate belief that this limited practitioner creativity or ignored practitioner expertise. We will address that misconception later in this chapter.

   Facts. Reviewed in chapter three, the *process of evidence-based practice* specifically includes a step in which the practitioner reviews possible interventions with the client. In the IOM description (2001), step four in the *process of evidence-based practice* specifies that relevant evidence about interventions should be integrated with the practitioner's clinical expertise, client values, and circumstances (Institute of Medicine, 2001). In Gambrill's descriptions of the *process of evidence-based practice* in social work, she emphasizes that the practitioner should discuss evidence-based interventions with their client so that based upon their values and circumstance, the client may make an informed choice of which to use (Gambrill, 1999, 2010, 2018). The same emphasis is embedded within definitions articulated by the American Psychological Association (2006).

   In fact, throughout the phases of engagement, assessment, planning, intervention, and evaluation, there are many client choice points in *evidence-based practice models*. Collaborative treatment models specifically require that clients be engaged as full partners in defining problems, determining goals, contributing to assessment, as well as in shaping, selecting, and evaluating interventions. Addis, Wade, and Hatgis (1999) provide suggestions for strategies to ensure client voice within evidence-based models.

Misconception: The Cookbook Myth

This near-mythical misconception stems from the requirement that *evidence-based practice models* should have a written description of participants, elements, activities, and phases of treatment. This clearly differentiates *evidence-based practice models* from eclectic practice. Those who are most comfortable with an eclectic approach believed that written manuals, protocols, or guidelines diminish or ignore practitioner expertise and creativity (Gitterman & Knight, 2013; Wampold, 2001; Wampold & Bhati, 2004).

   Facts. Written manuals, protocols, or guidelines simply provide a framework or principles of practice and proven strategies. As any good cook will tell you, whether baking a cake or preparing a meal, in implementing a proven recipe, the baker's or chef's actions depend upon their knowledge, experience, judgment, and skill as they adjust to contextual factors. For example, a recipe may suggest more time in mixing chocolate, but on a sweltering day, an experienced chef may limit time exposure to the heat and use refrigeration to help cool the mixture.

This is also true in behavioral health care and social services. In implementing treatment guidelines, the practitioner's actions depend on their knowledge and experience, their judgment and skill, and their assessment of contextual factors. Practitioner expertise and style shape client engagement, assessment/exploration of contributing factors to problems, as well as delivery of interventions. Furthermore, client choice points in *evidence-based practice models* ensure that the practice model is not delivered as a cookbook approach to complex issues. Finally, when challenges arise in treatment, the practice guidelines provide a compass, not a detailed roadmap to help the practitioner refocus and redirect their expertise.

Misconception: The Therapeutic Alliance

This misconception may be the most frequently asserted. In early debates about evidence-based practice, critics asserted that the therapeutic alliance, the clients' trust and ability to work with the practitioner, was the most important factor contributing to improved outcomes. They opined that manuals for evidence-based treatments overlook this alliance which is frequently cited as a predictor of positive outcomes in psychodynamic counseling (Wampold & Bhati, 2004; Wampold, 2001). Characterized as a relationship of support and trust, or sometimes as collaborative development of goals and objectives between client and practitioner, these studies suggest that in such counseling, this alliance contributes more to outcomes than do practitioner techniques (Ardito & Rabellino, 2011). Such criticisms erroneously asserted that written protocols did not emphasize establishing trust and a working relationship between practitioner and client. Some of the critics later joined proponents of the *common factors framework* and asserted that the therapeutic alliance, client motivation, and practitioner factors are responsible for treatment outcomes to a greater extent than are the elements and activities described in protocols for *evidence-based practice models* (Duncan, Miller, Wampold, & Hubble, 2010; Sparks & Muro, 2009).

Facts. Engaging client trust and creating a working relationship is both an initial phase (engagement) and a persistent element across *evidence-based treatment models* and in a *process of evidence-based practice*. Further, in psychodynamic and eclectic approaches to practice, when the client does not trust or engage, it is described as client resistance, whereas the accountability for client engagement and development of a working relationship clearly rests with practitioners and treatment teams in collaborative evidence-based practice models (Hengeller et al., 2009; Linehan, Cochran, & Kehrer, 2001).

Misconception: Staff Discomfort

Critics of evidence-based practice sometimes raise concerns that staff will be uncomfortable if the service organization adopts an *evidence-based practice model*. Practitioners, supervisors, and other staffs may be accustomed to applying an eclectic approach or may not be comfortable with data-informed coaching and measures of fidelity. This concern states the obvious. Change in accustomed activities can at first be uncomfortable. More importantly, it ignores the ethical responsibilities of the organization and the practitioner to deliver the best possible treatment to clients.

Facts. There is a rich literature reflected in discussions about a *process of evidence-based practice* that we have previously described. Practitioners and organizations can approach engagement, assessment, planning, interventions, and evaluation of evidence-based practices without the agency selecting a single practice model.

For example, in Houston's Children's Mental Health Initiative grant site, elements from two *evidence-based practice models* were integrated with elements and activities of a wraparound approach. This included Solution-Based Casework's use of timelines in thinking through the family life cycle, and use of MST fit circle multisystemic assessment to design behavioral interventions. With concurrent adjustments to training, coaching and case data forms, over 18 months, these adjustments improved wraparound fidelity above the national mean and improved youth academic and behavioral outcomes (Bertram, Schaffer, & Charnin, 2014).

As we reviewed in Chap. 3, some authors suggest a *common elements approach* (Barth et al., 2012), in which practitioners learn similar elements from proven or promising practices for use in different phases of service delivery. Also, Motivational Interviewing (Miller & Rollnick, 2012) is a proven practice frequently used in engagement, assessment, and planning with clients that complements the application of other treatments such as Trauma-Focused Cognitive Behavioral Therapy (Cohen, Mannarino, & Deblinger, 2006) in planning and intervention phases of service delivery.

Misconception: Staff Marketability and Turnover

Although this misconception emerged in early debates about evidence-based practice, it is still asserted as a concern to this day. Some believe that by investing in training and coaching a practitioner, supervisor, or other staffs to deliver an evidence-based practice, the organization makes them more marketable. Thus, staff turnover may increase as they pursue other employment opportunities. Interestingly, this concern implicitly assumes other organizations may be adopting that evidence-based practice. This misconception or concern also ignores the organization's ethical responsibility to deliver the best possible treatment to its clients.

Facts. Many organizational factors influence staff turnover, and salary, benefits, workload, and organizational culture are consistently identified as primary factors

(Aarons & Sawitzky, 2006). Through the research establishing efficacy and effectiveness, many *evidence-based treatment models* identify optimal practitioner workload capacity (Henggeler et al., 2009; Alexander et al., 1998). Furthermore, because elements, activities and, phases of the practice model, as well as its coaching and supervision, workload and use of data to guide implementation are identified, confusion about expectations, roles, and responsibilities can be diminished. This contributes to a more cohesive, supportive organizational culture. In fact, in a state children's service system, implementation of evidence-based practice that included fidelity monitoring and supportive consultation predicted lower staff turnover rates (Aarons, Sommerfeld, Hecht, Silovsky, & Chaffin, 2009).

Misconception: Too Expensive

An early and frequently stated opinion about *evidence-based treatment models* was that they were too costly for agencies, schools, or programs to implement. This belief was usually asserted without actual facts of how much it might cost to contract with a practice model purveyor to provide training, coaching, or data systems to support staff development and the effective delivery of the treatment model with fidelity. As we approach the end of the second decade of the twenty-first century, this opinion or belief has less valence.

Facts. Some *evidence-based practice models*, like Multisystemic Therapy (MST), focus upon more complex behavioral problems and therefore require ongoing technical and clinical support. While the initial investment for some evidence-based models may seem more costly than less proven practices, the evidence-based models produce long-term cost savings through lower rates of recidivism.

We reviewed several definitions for and repositories of evidence-based models in Chap. 3. Cost-benefit analysis and sustainment of treatment outcomes are key elements for the most thoroughly proven practices. We provide a sample of resources at the end of this book with links to sites such as the Washington State Institute for Public Policy, Blueprints for Healthy Youth Development, and the California Clearinghouse for Evidence-Based Practice in Child Welfare that provide cost-benefit analysis of evidence-based practice models.

Major funding sources like the Children's Bureau now require the use of proven practices (see review of Family First Prevention Services Act in Chap. 3) and even provide time and financial support to install the practice model before beginning to implement it.

Misconception: Promoted by Insurance Companies to Cut Costs

The juxtaposition or concurrence of this opinion or belief with the previous one should intrigue our astute readers. During the early debates about evidence-based practice, proponents of eclectic practice sometimes asserted the opinion that evidence-based practice was part of strategies used by insurance companies to cut their costs. Let's briefly ponder this concern. It assumes that insurance companies do not wish to overpay or to pay as little as possible for client treatment. No doubt, this is true. It is indeed a key pillar of capitalism. This opinion or belief may also assume that limiting costs will restrict client access to services.

Fact. Although capitalism cannot change without significant legislation or social upheaval, we can shed the bright light of facts upon this misconception. Insurance provider's support for evidence-based practice models directs funds to interventions with a greater likelihood of efficiently improving client outcomes. As a result, more clients have access to proven practice models, and recidivism of behaviors of concern is lower when clients participate in evidence-based treatment. Therefore, their quality of life improves. In this case, benefits are incurred across the system. For example, a study of one evidence-based intervention that is often critiqued as being quite expensive to implement found that within a statewide implementation of Multisystemic Therapy in New Mexico, in addition to superior clinical outcomes across a range of domains and cost savings in multiple systems (e.g., juvenile justice and child welfare), Medicaid itself saved $1.35 for every $1 invested (Dopp et al., 2018).

Misconception: No Evidence-Based Case Management Practices

We have heard this belief stated by persons representing organizations that rely upon case management to address their clientele's diverse needs. We have also heard it asserted by social work faculty who are responsible for developing graduates who become practitioners, supervisors, managers, and administrators in these organizations. Professional degree programs play an indirect, yet key role in shaping selection and implementation of services. We will examine curricula for workforce preparation in Chap. 5.

Fact. There are at least two evidence-based case management practice models, Assertive Community Treatment and Solution-Based Casework. Both emphasize collaborative, culturally competent engagement of client/family voice in shaping assessments, planning, and interventions, as well as in evaluation of interventions and outcomes. There is also a growing body of evidence supporting wraparound care coordination as a research-based practice, and it is being taught in some social work curricula (Bertram, Charnin, Kerns, & Long, 2015; Bruns, 2008; Bruns, Pullmann, Sather, Brinson, & Ramey, 2015; Suter & Bruns, 2008).

References

Aarons, G. A., & Sawitzky, A. C. (2006). Organizational culture and climate and mental health provider attitudes toward evidence-based practice. *Psychological Services, 3*(1), 61.

Aarons, G. A., Sommerfeld, D., Hecht, D., Silovsky, J., & Chaffin, M. (2009). The impact of evidence-based practice implementation and fidelity monitoring on staff turnover: Evidence for a protective effect. *Journal of Consulting and Clinical Psychology, 77*(2), 270–280.

Addis, M., Wade, W. A., & Hatgis, C. (1999). Barriers to dissemination of evidence-based practices: Addressing practitioners' concerns about manual-based psychotherapies. *Clinical Psychology: Science and Practice, 6*, 430–441.

Alexander, J., Barton, C., Gordon, D., Grotpeter, J., Hansson, K., Harrison, R., et al. (1998). *Blueprints for violence prevention, book three: Functional family therapy.* Boulder: Center for the Study and Prevention of Violence.

American Psychological Association Presidential Task Force on Evidence Based-Practice. (2006). Evidence-based practice in psychology. *American Psychologist, 61*(4), 271–285.

Ardito, R. B., & Rabellino, D. (2011). Therapeutic alliance and outcome of psychotherapy: Historical excursus, measurements, and prospects for research. *Frontiers in Psychology, 2,* 270.

Barth, R. P., Lee, B. R., Lindsey, M. A., Collins, K. S., Strieder, F., Chorpita, B. F., et al. (2012). Evidence-based practice at a crossroads: The timely emergence of common elements and common factors. *Research on Social Work Practice, 22*(1), 108–119.

Bertram, R. M., Charnin, L. A., Kerns, S. E. U., & Long, A. C. (2015). Evidence-based practices in North American MSW curricula. *Research on Social Work Practice, 25*(6), 737–748.

Bertram, R. M., Schaffer, P., & Charnin, L. (2014). Changing organization culture: Data driven participatory evaluation and revision of wraparound implementation. *Journal of Evidence-Based Social Work, 11,* 18–29.

Bruns, E. J. (2008). The evidence base and wraparound. In E. J. Bruns & J. S. Walker (Eds.), *The resource guide to wraparound.* Portland: National Wraparound Initiative, Research and Training Center for Family Support and Children's Mental Health.

Bruns, E. J., Pullmann, M. D., Sather, A., Brinson, R. D., & Ramey, M. (2015). Effectiveness of wraparound versus case management for children and adolescents: Results of a randomized study. *Administration and Policy in Mental Health and Mental Health Services Research, 42*(3), 309–322.

Chambless, D. L., & Ollendick, T. H. (2001). Empirically supported psychological interventions: Controversies and evidence. *Annual Review of Psychology, 52,* 685–716.

Cohen, J. A., Mannarino, A. P., & Deblinger, E. (2006). *Treating trauma and traumatic grief in children and adolescents.* Guilford Publications.

Dopp, A. R., Coen, A. S., Smith, A. B., Reno, J., Bernstein, D. H., Kerns, S. E. U., et al. (2018). Economic impact of the statewide implementation of an evidence-based treatment: Multisystemic therapy in New Mexico. *Behavior Therapy, 49*(4), 551–566.

Duncan, B. L., Miller, S. D., Wampold, B. E., & Hubble, M. A. (2010). *The heart and soul of change: Delivering what works* (2nd ed.). Washington, DC: American Psychological Association.

Gambrill, E. (1999). Evidence-based practice: An alternative to authority-based practice. *Families in Society: The Journal of Contemporary Human Services, 80,* 341–350.

Gambrill, E. (2010). Evidence-informed practice: Antidote to propaganda in the helping profession. *Research on Social Work Practice, 20,* 302–320.

Gambrill, E. (2018). Contributions of the process of evidence-based practice to implementation: Educational opportunities. *Journal of Social Work Education, 54*(sup1), S113–S125.

Gitterman, A., & Knight, C. (2013). Evidence-guided practice: Integrating the science and art of social work. *Families in Society: The Journal of Contemporary Social Services, 94,* 70–78.

Henggeler, S. W., Rowland, M. D., Randall, J., Ward, D. M., Pickrel, S. G., Cunningham, P. B., ... & Santos, A. B. (1999). Home-based multisystemic therapy as an alternative to the hospitalization of youths in psychiatric crisis: Clinical outcomes. *Journal of the American Academy of Child & Adolescent Psychiatry, 38*(11), 1331–1339.

Henggeler, S. W., Schoenwald, S. K., Borduin, C. M., Rowland, M. D., & Cunningham, P. B. (2009). *Multisystemic therapy for anti-social behavior in children and adolescents* (2nd ed.). New York: Guilford Press.

Huey, S. J., Jr., & Polo, A. J. (2008). Evidence-based psychosocial treatments for ethnic minority youth. *Journal of Clinical Child & Adolescent Psychology, 37*(1), 262–301.

Institute of Medicine. (2001). *Crossing the quality chasm: A new healthy system for the 21st century.* Washington, DC: National Academic Press.

Letourneau, E. J., Henggeler, S. W., Borduin, C. M., Schewe, P. A., McCart, M. R., Chapman, J. E., et al. (2009). Multisystemic therapy for juvenile sexual offenders: 1-year results from a randomized effectiveness trial. *Journal of Family Psychology, 23,* 89–102.

Linehan, M. M., Cochran, B. N., & Kehrer, C. A. (2001). Dialectical behavior therapy for borderline personality disorder. In D. H. Barlow (Ed.), *Clinical handbook of psychological disorders: A step-by-step treatment manual* (3rd ed., pp. 470–522). New York, NY: Guilford Press.

Miller, W. R., & Rollnick, S. (2012). *Motivational interviewing: Helping people change.* Guilford Press.

Nowak, C., & Heinrichs, N. (2008). A comprehensive meta-analysis of Triple P-Positive Parenting Program using hierarchical linear modeling: Effectiveness and moderating variables. *Clinical Child and Family Psychology Review, 11*(3), 114.

Sparks, J. A., & Muro, M. L. (2009). Client-directed wraparound: The client as connector in community collaboration. *Journal of Systemic Therapies, 28,* 63–76.

Straus, S. E., & McAlister, F. A. (2000). Evidence-based medicine: A commentary on common criticisms. *Canadian Medical Association Journal, 163*(7), 837–841.

Suter, J. C., & Bruns, E. J. (2008). *A narrative review of wraparound outcome studies. Resource guide to wraparound.* Portland, OR: National Wraparound Initiative, Research and Training Center for Family Support and Children's Mental Health.

Swenson, C. C., Schaeffer, C. M., Henggeler, S. W., Faldowski, R., & Mayhew, A. M. (2010). Multisystemic therapy for child abuse and neglect: A randomized effectiveness trial. *Journal of Family Psychology, 24,* 497–507.

Trupin, E. J., Kerns, S. E. U., Walker, S. C., DeRobertis, M. T., & Stewart, D. G. (2011). Family integrated transitions: A promising program for juvenile offenders with co-occurring disorders. *Journal of Child & Adolescent Substance Abuse, 20*(5), 421–436.

Wampold, B. (2001). *The great psychotherapy debate.* Mahwah, NJ: Lawrence Erlbaum.

Wampold, B. E., & Bhati, K. S. (2004). Attending to the omissions: A historical examination of evidence-based practice movements. *Professional Psychology: Research and Practice, 35,* 563–570.

Webb, S. A. (2001). Some considerations on the validity of evidence-based practice in social work. *British Journal of Social Work, 31*(1), 57–79.

Chapter 5
Workforce Preparation: Academic Curricula and Concerns

Despite an increasing emphasis on utilizing a *process of evidence-based practice* or *evidence-supported treatment models* (Chambless & Hollon, 1998; Kazdin, Bass, Ayers, & Rodgers, 1990), a gap between what we know works and what we actually do still characterizes much of social work, marriage, and family therapy, and behavioral health care (Bruns, Kerns, Pullmann, Hensley, Lutterman & Hoagwood, 2015). Curriculum development and instruction in professional degree programs contribute to this research-to-practice gap (Bertram, Charnin, Kerns, & Long, 2015; Drabick & Goldfried, 2000; Cannata, Marlowe, Bertram, Kerns, Wolf, & Choi; Owenz & Hall, 2011). Curricula are developed by faculty and reviewed and approved (or not) by faculty committees. Hence, *faculty concerns or misconceptions, their knowledge and experience are critical factors that may support, slow, or impede the integration of evidence-based practice and implementation science into academic curricula.*

Faculty concerns were reflected in and fueled by the early definitional debates we reviewed in Chap. 3. These concerns were fueled by misconceptions we reviewed in Chap. 4. Was evidence-based practice a process that practitioners should use and individualize with every client to select evidence-based interventions? Or was evidence-based practice a specific treatment model with a clear description of its elements and activities and how they improved client outcomes (theory of change) that was tested with well-defined client populations in randomized controlled assignment trials? Could both be true? Thyer and Myers (2011) offered a deep historical analysis of the emergence of evidence-based practice in social work and related disciplines. They differentiate a process of evidence-based social work practice from empirically supported treatment models. To begin this chapter, we discuss how social work and related disciplines grappled with the relationship between science and practice in workforce preparation.

© Springer Nature Switzerland AG 2019
R. Bertram and S. Kerns, *Selecting and Implementing Evidence-Based Practice*,
https://doi.org/10.1007/978-3-030-11325-4_5

Marriage and Family Therapy

Pre-dating debates about evidence-based practice, the American Psychological Association articulated the Boulder scientist–practitioner model which stated that to be effective practitioners, students should be trained in both clinical practice and in research. (Frank, 1984; Raimy, 1950). Karam and Sprenkle (2010) suggested this approach might not be effective for marriage and family therapy master's degree students whose career ambitions were not focused on research. Instead, they proposed developing a *research-informed* perspective that maintains a clinical focus informed by research. In this approach, marriage and family therapy academic programs could integrate the Council on American Marriage and Family Therapy Education's (COAMFTE) required academic courses on historical and theoretical roots of family-centered empirically supported treatments.

The efficacy of the scientist–practitioner model and the research-informed approach was recently compared in a quasi-experimental study of 68 students at accredited marriage and family therapy programs (Meyer, Templeton, Stinson, & Codone, 2016). Results suggested that students in courses promoting either a scientist–practitioner or a research-informed focus demonstrated significant improvements in knowledge of both clinical and research competencies. No significant differences were found between the two approaches. However, despite requirements to incorporate research and evaluation into curricula, students did not demonstrate increased knowledge and skills in evidence-based practices (Meyer et al., 2016). These authors suggest a more targeted and directive approach is needed to improve evidence-based practice competencies. Recent COAMFTE standards require programs to "infuse a culture of research and establish the importance of research-based education within the profession" (COAMFTE, 2017, p. 4). Programs must now establish the level of emphasis they will place on research within their mission and then adhere to those standards (COAMFTE, 2017).

Given its origins in family systems theory, Oka and Whiting (2013) asserted that to bridge the science-to-practice gap in marriage and family therapy, systemic research should focus upon process, dyadic, and sequential analysis. Stith (2014) asserted that to bridge the research to practice gap, marriage and family therapy programs must increase expectations for students to engage in rigorous research. However, a review of *Journal of Marital and Family Therapy* articles published between 2005 and 2015 noted that although the number of research articles increased, the percentage of articles presenting quantitative research had not (Parker, Chang, & Thomas, 2016).

Social Work

In 2008, the Council on Social Work Education (CSWE) accreditation standards first included the expectation that social workers "apply evidence-based interventions, evaluate their practice, and use research findings to improve both practice and policy."

CSWE's more recent accreditation standards (2015) continued this emphasis and provided specific guidelines that require students to engage in research to evaluate their own practice, as well as to learn specific evidence-based interventions (CSWE, 2015). In that year, an Institute of Medicine report (2015) specifically identified the need for social work and psychology to provide effective training in evidence-based practices, as the exiting Director of the National Institute of Health asserted that professional credentialing standards must require mastery of such practices (Insel, 2015).

> *Despite such continuing encouragement and guidance, the wheel of change turns slowly in academia where faculty determine curricula focus and content. What faculty know or don't know, what they can or cannot do, as well as their opinions and beliefs shape academic and field curricula.*
>
> *Logically, in addition to a profession's values and ethics, advances in science, expectations of funding sources and the related needs of service systems and organizations should inform curricula focus and content.*

Workforce Readiness

At the 2002 Georgetown Summer Institutes, participants who shared interests in evidence-based and promising practices for children, youth, and families discussed the disparate ways these practices were unfolding across North America. As the evidence-based practice debates described in Chap. 3 unfolded, a group of research and teaching faculty from a variety of disciplines, as well as behavioral healthcare administrators and practitioners and evidence-based practice purveyors formed the Child and Family Evidence-Based Practice Consortium in 2004 to collaborate, support, and learn from each other (Kanary, Bertram, & Bernstein, 2017).

In the ensuing decade, contributors to Consortium projects focused on workforce readiness. Notably, a Canadian participant from the University of Toronto published an examination of the readiness of newly hired master's level clinicians to conduct evidence-based practice (Barwick, 2011). She surveyed 589 administrators and supervisors from North American behavioral healthcare programs who were responsible for hiring child and family practitioners who had earned master's level professional degrees (most earned a social work degree).

Survey respondents indicated that basic abilities necessary for evidence-based practice were often not well developed in those professional degree programs. These included the ability to formulate a clinical question about the behavior(s) of concern, to search primary or secondary sources or repositories of research on evidence-based practices, and to critically review this literature to select an appropriate intervention and evaluate its effectiveness upon delivery.

> *The abilities evaluated in Barwick's study (2011) support **the process of evidence-based practice** presented in Chap. 3. We'll discuss each of these abilities as we review related studies in this chapter.*

Of the 589 responding administrators and supervisors, most (69%) believed that the ability to formulate a clinical question, identify and apply an intervention and evaluate the outcomes was an essential competency for evidence-based practice. However, 64% of the respondents indicated this was not an ability that master's level practitioners demonstrated upon hire. Most respondents (56%) also indicated that the ability to critically review research in professional literature was necessary to select and deliver an evidence-based practice, but 55% of the respondents indicated the newly hired master's level practitioners were not able to do so. Finally, 43% of the respondents believed that the ability to search sources for professional literature was integral to providing evidence-based practice but 54% of the 589 respondents indicated these abilities were not evident in their newly hired master's level practitioners (Barwick, 2011).

Results of this large survey clearly suggested that most newly hired master's level practitioners had not developed necessary knowledge and skills to provide evidence-based practice. These abilities then had to be developed by the behavioral healthcare programs in on-the-job training and coaching. Respondents were also asked about the extent to which their behavioral healthcare program collaborated with academic programs to discuss workforce preparation and readiness (Barwick, 2011). Only 25% of the 589 respondents indicated this occurred, while 36% said it did not, and 39% were uncertain. Most respondents that indicated there was contact between their behavioral healthcare organization and graduate degree programs reported the purpose of contact was to secure practicum placements, while only 16% reported that they made curriculum recommendations, and only 2% suggested course assignments (Barwick, 2011).

These results prompted a number of Child and Family Evidence-Based Practice Consortium participants to explore the extent to which evidence-based practice was taught in MSW curricula (Bertram, Charnin, Kerns, & Long, 2015) and in master's level marriage and family therapy programs (Cannata, Marlowe, et al., in progress). Both studies queried deans and directors of these master's level programs using similar surveys as well as the same questions posed in the Barwick (2011) study. The studies also explored respondents' perspectives on both the barriers and the implications of teaching evidence-based practice.

Evidence-Based Practice in MSW Curricula

Deans or directors of 215 MSW programs in the USA and Canada received the survey and 58 programs responded via a secure Web site, representing a 27% response rate. As in the Barwick (2011) study, this examination of MSW curricula used the classic criteria for an evidence-based practice model: a clearly defined target population, written elements, activities and phases of practice, and research supporting its effectiveness with that population established in random-assignment control group studies (Chambless & Ollendick, 2001; Silverman & Hinshaw, 2008). Fifty-two of the responding programs (90%) reported (sometimes not accurately) that they taught practices that met these criteria. A total of 163 practices were identified as meeting these criteria. However, upon careful review of the literature by the study team and one outside reviewer ($n = 5$), only 108 of these practices (66%) met study criteria (99% inter-rater reliability).

To examine the extent to which these practices were taught, this study focused through a framework of intervention components identified by the National Implementation Research Network (Bertram, Blase, & Fixsen, 2015; Fixsen, Blase, Naoom, & Wallace, 2009; Fixsen, Naoom, Blase, Friedman, & Wallace, 2005). These included whether research supporting its effectiveness with a specific population was taught, as well as the practice model's activities, elements and phases, the theory base(s) supporting this, and its theory of change. Responding deans and directors reported that for 89 of those 108 practice models, all four intervention components were presented to students and that this included opportunity to apply the practice in assignments or in their field practicum. Motivational Interviewing, Cognitive Behavioral Therapies, and Solution-Focused models were more commonly taught than family-centered models such as Multisystemic Therapy, Functional Family Therapy, or Structural Family Therapy.

> *Although MSW graduates are frequently employed in case management positions, evidence-based practices such as Solution-Based Casework and Assertive Community Treatment were rarely taught in responding programs.*

Who teaches these practices? Academic programs are diminishing the number of full-time faculty and replacing them with adjunct faculty who are not offered benefits and whose salaries are significantly less than full-time faculty (Bettinger & Long, 2010). In this study, most of the evidence-based practices were taught by adjunct faculty (Bertram et al., 2015). *However, it is the full-time and tenured or tenure track faculty that develop the focus of curricula and the courses taught by these adjuncts.*

Barriers to teaching these practices. All 58 responding MSW program deans or directors identified barriers to teaching specific evidence-based practices. *Seven identified field learning sites as a barrier because those sites used case management or eclectic approaches to practice.* Twenty-four programs indicated that Council on Social Work Education curriculum requirements left little room for adding specific practice models into their academic courses. These responses suggested that programs were not considering integrating a process of evidence-based practice across the curriculum as the Brown School of Social Work has accomplished at Washington University in St. Louis (Howard, McMillen, & Pollio, 2003; Proctor, 2007).

The next set of barriers echo the early debates about evidence-based practice and the misconceptions that fueled them. Twenty-six programs identified faculty confusion or differences about definitions of evidence-based practice as a barrier. Many of the concerns, opinions, beliefs, and misconceptions we reviewed in Chaps. 3 and 4 of this book were voiced, including the perceived restrictiveness of the classic criteria defining an evidence-based practice (Chambless & Ollendick, 2001; Silverman & Hinshaw, 2008). Some respondents indicated that faculty-believed evidence-based treatments were "not a good fit" for minority populations or that they were developed only for "specific diagnosable problems." Astute readers will note how these responses reflect common misconceptions about evidence-based practices reviewed in Chap. 4.

None of the respondents noted the emergence of more expansive definitions and criteria reviewed in Chap. 3 of this book. No program identified the debate about whether evidence-based practice should be taught as a process or as specific treatment models as a barrier.

By far the most commonly identified barrier ($n = 37$) to teaching specific evidence-based practices was the program's faculty. Twelve programs identified limitations in faculty knowledge and experience. Eight identified barriers resulting from faculty members' theoretical orientation and associated beliefs that evidence-based treatment models were too structured or their beliefs that they were a cookbook approach that limited "the art of therapy" and practitioner creativity. This was especially true if the faculty member embraced psychodynamic theory or holistic, eclectic practice. Interestingly, one respondent stated that such perspectives may be the result of designing courses and curricula for private practice rather than the reality that most graduates work in organizations that increasingly are required by funding sources to provide evidence-based practices.

Positive implications. Respondents noted 90 different positive implications for MSW programs teaching evidence-based practice. Most noted that this improved the credibility of the social work profession ($n = 19$), by improving client outcomes ($n = 10$), or by improving access to funds ($n = 5$). Nineteen responses coalesced around workforce readiness including knowledge and skill development.

Scientific approach to practice. In Barwick's study (2011), 69% of the 589 responding behavioral healthcare program administrators and supervisors believed a scientific approach was important for effective evidence-based practice. However, 64% reported that master's level practitioners did not demonstrate this ability which then had to be developed through on-the-job training and coaching. In the MSW curriculum study (Bertram, Charnin, et al., 2015), 69% of the 58 responding academic programs reported they thoroughly or extensively developed this ability in their students.

Search skills. In Barwick's study (2011), 43% of the 589 responding behavioral healthcare program administrators and supervisors believed that the ability to search, find, and use reliable sources about specific evidence-based practices was important for practitioner effectiveness, while 54% reported that upon hire, master's level practitioners did not demonstrate this ability. Only 35% of the responding academic programs in the MSW curriculum study reported that their program thoroughly or extensively sought to develop this ability in their students.

Critical appraisal skills. In Barwick's study (2011), 56% of the 589 responding behavioral healthcare administrators and supervisors believed that the ability to critically appraise research findings was necessary in effective evidence-based practice. However, 55% of respondents indicated practitioners with master degrees did not possess these skills and had to develop them on the job. In the MSW curriculum study, 67% of responding MSW programs believed they thoroughly or extensively addressed critical appraisal skills.

Findings from the MSW curriculum study prompted the Child and Family Evidence-Based Practice Consortium to develop a series of four national webinars for social work faculty. Webinar contributors from several academic programs addressed misconceptions with facts and shared how their programs integrated evidence-based practice, and implementation science in specific courses, as well as how the George Warren Brown School of Social Work integrated the process of evidence-based practice across academic and field curricula. These webinars are available at https://ebpconsortium.com/webinars/msw-faculty-webinars/. Participants in the webinars suggested a special issue of the *Journal of Social Work Education* focusing on how to integrate implementation science and evidence-based practice in both academic and field curricula. That special issue is discussed in the final chapter of this book.

Marriage and Family Therapy Curricula

While developing and presenting those webinars for social work faculty, Consortium participants initiated a study of evidence-based practice in marriage and family therapy (MFT) curricula. Based upon Chambless and Ollendick (2001) and Silverman and Hinshaw (2008), this study applied the same criteria for defining an evidence-based practice as was used in the MSW curriculum study (Bertram, Charnin, et al., 2015), and in Barwick's investigation (2011). An evidence-based practice had a clearly defined target population; written elements, activities, and phases of service delivery; and research supporting effectiveness with that population established through random-assignment control group studies. Electronic surveys and telephone interviews resulted in 27 of the 89 accredited master's degree programs in marriage and family therapy responding (30% response rate). Thirty-seven practice models were identified as an evidence-based practice that met study criteria (Kerns, Bertram, et al., in progress).

A majority of programs taught specific *evidence-based treatment models* ($n = 23$; 85%). Unlike the MSW curriculum study, tenure track faculty were more likely to teach these practice models than other faculty, and the MFT programs were smaller and did not rely upon adjunct faculty as much as the MSW programs. Specifically, 85% of full professors, 61% of associate professors, and 70% of assistant professors taught evidence-based treatments, compared with 46% of non-tenure track instructors and 45% of adjunct faculty. The EBPs most commonly taught included Cognitive Behavioral Therapy, Emotion-Focused Therapy, Functional Family Therapy, and Multisystemic Therapy.

Advantages for students. In the MFT curriculum study, the most frequently identified benefit was that teaching evidence-based practice prepared students for employment by developing literacy about the field, as well as clinical skills ($n = 12$; 44%;). Several respondents stated this creates better clinicians by providing clarity about practice, which increases student confidence, and makes them more marketable.

Advantages for the profession. Ten respondents (37%) believed marriage and family practitioners should be able to demonstrate that their practice is effective, and that this increased the credibility of the profession. One of these respondents specifically stated that this provides credibility to a field that is often perceived as an art and not a science. Two of these respondents believed it was beneficial to have a strong research base to demonstrate that marriage and family therapy can be more effective than other approaches, while one highlighted that knowledge of evidence-based practice can help secure research funding and insurance reimbursement.

Advantages for clients. Interestingly and quite similar to the MSW curriculum study, only a few programs discussed benefits for clients. Three MFT programs noted that teaching what works is essential to meet specific client needs. One respondent believed that as a result, graduates were more focused on client context.

Barriers to teaching EBPs. Similar to the MSW curriculum study, faculty misconceptions or beliefs were identified as a barrier by the majority of respondents ($n = 17$; 62%). Ten of these respondents (37%) believed that evidence-based practices were too narrow in their focus. Some believed that the specific treatment models were not studied with a diverse client population, or did not consider the complexity or uniqueness of individuals, or could not be applied in private practice or small treatment settings. Several noted that simply because there is (or is not) research supporting effectiveness of an intervention does not mean a treatment is better (or worse).

Another frequently cited barrier was that many MFT faculty are not trained in evidence-based treatments ($n = 13$; 48%). This was attributed to the aging of faculty, the small number of faculty, or to faculty not being currently engaged in clinical practice. Time was a related challenge associated with developing new clinical knowledge and abilities or to faculty understanding newer treatment models. Several respondents noted that senior faculty who are unfamiliar with newer *evidence-based practice models* often present bias and barriers when the program considers integrating evidence-based practice in the curricula.

Many respondents identified a lack of room in the curriculum to include content on evidence-based treatment models ($n = 15$; 55%). Similar to programs that did not teach evidence-based practice, these respondents discussed how COAMFTE accreditation standards and licensing requirements determined course content leaving little time or space for presenting *evidence-based treatment models*. Several respondents associated this challenge with having smaller programs and few faculty available to present the required content. As a result, when *evidence-based treatment models* were taught, they could only present overviews of select models.

Of particular interest, nine respondents (33%) believed that evidence-based treatment was not aligned with MFT values or with the theoretical orientation of the program. Some believed these practices were more individually focused and not sufficiently focused on couples, families, or relational issues or complexities. One respondent explained that the main focus of their program is on the person of the practitioner as the most important ingredient of the therapeutic relationship, and that this transcends any model's effectiveness. One respondent did not want to tell students that they have to practice in a certain way. Another stated that their program did not teach students manualized approaches, especially if some entity was profiting from the approach.

Other beliefs identified as barriers reflected misconceptions discussed in Chap. 4 of this book, including explicit criticisms about randomized control trials, cautions about the validity of some findings, and concerns that teaching manualized treatments would limit clinician flexibility. One rather odd theme identified by three programs was their perception that students are not ready to learn about or to use evidence-based treatments. These respondents believed students did not have the ability to understand research because as clinicians, they are just learning to engage clients.

Of the four responding programs (14%) that did not teach evidence-based practice, two identified logistics as the primary barrier (too little room in the curriculum, competing demands, and untrained faculty). The other two programs noted multiple concerns, including a belief that students would become sure and certain, rather than curious and considering, "thus becoming skilled workers rather than healers."

Comparison of Studies

For comparison with the Barwick (2011) and the MSW curriculum studies (Bertram, Charnin, et al., 2015), the same three questions asked how well the MFT program developed student skill sets that support evidence-based practice. This included scientific approach, search, and critical appraisal skills. As in those studies, a scientific approach was defined as the ability to formulate a clinical problem, develop or utilize the appropriate intervention strategy, and evaluate service delivery for outcomes. Search skills were defined as knowledge of secondary sources of reliable information about evidence-based programs or promising practices. Critical appraisal skills were defined as the ability to accurately appraise research findings for validity, impact, and applicability and to draw on clinical expertise to integrate this knowledge with client information.

Scientific approach. In Barwick's study (2011), the majority (69%) of the responding behavioral health program administrators and supervisors identified this skill as necessary to effectively deliver an EBP. However, 64% of her respondents reported that master's level practitioners did not possess this skill set and had to develop it upon hire. In the MFT curriculum study, seventeen MFT programs (63%) indicated they thoroughly or extensively taught students a scientific approach to knowledge, while in the MSW curriculum study, 69% of responding academic programs reported they thoroughly or extensively developed this ability in their students (Bertram, Charnin, et al., 2015).

In the Barwick study (2011), most behavioral healthcare program administrators or supervisors believed this was an essential competency for evidence-based practice. In the MSW and MFT curriculum studies, most academic deans and directors believed their workforce preparation programs developed this ability in their master's level graduates. However, most administrators and supervisors in the Barwick study reported that newly hired master's level practitioners did not demonstrate this competency.

What is a scientific approach?

A scientific foundation for both knowledge and effective interventions begins with a clear description of the problem. It's important that the problem is specifically stated, or your search may lead you astray. For example, what are contributing factors or effective interventions with African American youth experiencing loss of appetite and depression?

The next step is to search for what is known. Access to university libraries or science-based search engines is critical. Simple strategies to maximize use of these tools will be discussed later in this chapter. However, finding information also requires evaluating its quality. How strong is the evidence? We reviewed emerging criteria in Chap. 3. These criteria should be understood by graduates of master's level professional degree programs.

Finally, your search for effective treatments may identify a practice that is not available in your community. We discuss how to address this in chaps. 8 and 9.

Search skills. In Barwick's (2011) study, this ability was identified as important for evidence-based practice by 43% of the responding behavioral healthcare program administrators and supervisors, and 54% of those respondents noted that newly hired master's level practitioners did not possess this skill upon hire. Only 35% of the responding MSW programs reported thoroughly or extensively developing this ability in their students, while 37% of responding MFT programs reported they thoroughly or extensively addressed student development of search skills and techniques.

Across the three studies, a majority of respondents reported that the ability to know where and how to search for information about effective practices was not well developed. Academic program responses suggest that a ***process of evidence-based practice*** was either not emphasized or was not well-supported.

Searching for relevant, peer-reviewed literature may seem daunting, especially when information from a myriad of Web sites and social media can be quickly accessed and reviewed. However, those sources may be of questionable quality and are often not science-based.

Searches for effective practices should be comprehensive. They are easily accessed via Web-based resources such as Cochrane Library, PubMed, Google Scholar, Web of Science, and PsycInfo. Search terms expand or limit the number of publications these sites identify.

Searching for effective practices usually begins with the behavior of concern. For example, in Chap 2, Tameisha's symptoms included loss of appetite and depression. Using Google Scholar and the term "loss of appetite" yields 631,000 results in .05 s. That's too many to be useful. But, by adding a client descriptor or additional behavior of concern to the search (e.g., "loss of appetite" "depression"), reduces the number of publications, and adding a third descriptor ("African American youth") reduces the number of possible publications to 162. In this example, each term is placed in quotations.

Titles and abstracts help identify useful publications. With those few particularly informative articles that emerge, it can be really helpful to do a reverse citation search. Google Scholar makes this easy. It identifies the number of publications that cited each article. By opening that link and reviewing those articles, more recent publications can be found. As an added bonus, Google Scholar also provides a hyperlink to related articles.

However, it may be even more time efficient to use a search engine that targets your particular interest and simultaneously identifies effective programs or practices. We offer some examples of program-specific databases in the Appendix to this book.

Critical appraisal skills. This was defined as the ability to accurately appraise research findings for validity, impact, and applicability to client characteristics. Barwick's 2011 study indicates that over half (56%) of the responding behavioral healthcare program administrators and supervisors perceived this as an essential skill to effectively deliver evidence-based practice, while 55% indicated that practitioners with master degrees did not possess this ability when they entered the workforce. Two-thirds of the MFT programs (66%) indicated they thoroughly or extensively addressed critical appraisal skills, while in the MSW curriculum study, 67% of responding MSW programs reported thoroughly or extensively addressing critical appraisal skills.

Similar to the scientific approach to effective practice, across the three studies, most program administrators or supervisors, and academic deans and directors believed this was an essential competency. But most administrators and supervisors in the Barwick study reported that newly hired master's level practitioners did not have this ability.

Critical appraisal skills are essential. To be blunt, sub-par research gets published. There can be substantial variability in the quality of studies. In addition to our Chap. 2 summary of Blueprints' criteria for evidence, here are a few guidelines.

Meta-analyses of literature on a practice or topic can be a valuable starting point because they explicitly identify a required standard of rigor in the examined studies.

Next best are studies that use random assignment with appropriate control groups (RCTs). The equivalence of subject characteristics between intervention and control groups should be considered. Could there be any potential bias that might differently impact the experimental or the control groups? In addition, were findings and analyses appropriate given the study design?

After RCTs, there are a host of quasi-experimental designs, some of which can be quite strong. Pre-post studies without control groups are a common but weaker means to establish evidence. These designs may be more common for behaviors in which identification of a control group is not feasible and within-subject designs are not appropriate.

Regardless of research design, a critique of the literature as it relates to the specific problem you are trying to address is essential. What was the population studied and how well does that match my client? How many people are represented in the studies (in general, smaller studies should be viewed as less generalizable than larger studies)? Did the researchers test for any mediators or moderators of effectiveness that might indicate that the intervention is more appropriate for some people than others? Were there other factors either noted or not addressed in the study that may influence program effectiveness (e.g., implementation factors)?

These three studies provide an interesting and mixed picture of the academic preparation of a capable, evidence-informed professional workforce. However, expectations of funding sources also shape workforce orientation and development. Using the Evidence-Based Practice Process Assessment Scale, Parrish and Rubin (2012) surveyed 865 social workers, psychologists, and licensed marriage and family therapists (LMFTs) in Texas about their orientation toward implementation of evidence-based practice. More recent MSW graduates had more favorable views of a ***process of evidence-based practice*** than less recent graduates, but psychologists with doctoral degrees reported greater orientation to implementing evidence-based practice than social workers and LMFTs who were more similar.

Summary

In developing curricula, any master's degree program necessarily must consider the context of organizations and the funding sources where their graduates will be employed. As articulated in Barwick's (2011) study, administrators and supervisors of behavioral healthcare programs reported that graduates were by and large not entering the workforce with the requisite knowledge and skills to deliver evidence-based practice in community-based behavioral health care.

As academic programs respond to accreditation requirements, they do so with a limited number of full-time faculty. Newer faculty may be more versed in specific *evidence-based treatment models*, while older faculty may lack such knowledge or may have theoretical differences, especially if they embrace psychodynamic theory and techniques or eclectic approaches to practice.

Most of the responding MFT programs that taught specific *evidence-based practice models* presented the elements and activities, theory base and theory of change, and the research supporting the practice model's effectiveness with specific populations. This thoroughness was less evident in MSW program responses. However, concerns about evidence-based practice were similar to those noted in the MSW curriculum study (Bertram, Charnin, et al., 2015).

It is wise to ponder what contributes to the persistence of these misconceptions. When we bring our child to a medical doctor, we expect and have confidence that the doctor follows tested guidelines for health or illness assessment and intervention. In behavioral health care, suggested guidelines for assessment and intervention exist in all forms of practice. Because evidence-based practices describe and test these guidelines, they should provide confidence for clients, practitioners, and educators.

Educators should thoroughly present an evidence-based practice model's core intervention components that include: (1) research supporting efficacy or effectiveness of the practice model with specific populations; (2) specification of key elements, participants, activities, and phases of the practice model; (3) the theory base(s) supporting this; and (4) the practice model's theory of change. They should also carefully examine how field learning sites support effective service delivery with fidelity. This should include understanding how the site selects, trains, and coaches staff, as well as the how data systems have been adjusted to evaluate fidelity and effectiveness of service delivery (Bertram, Choi, & Gillies, 2018; Bertram et al., 2015; Bertram, King, Pederson, & Nutt, 2014). A special issue of the *Journal of Social Work Education* (2018) offers ten examples of how social work programs are integrating implementation science and evidence-based practice in academic and field curricula. It is heartening to note that the call for papers for this special issue resulted in over 50 proposed manuscripts. In the final chapter of this book, we will review examples and suggest how programs can address faculty barriers to integrate both evidence-based practice and implementation science into both academic and field curricula.

> *Implementation science emerged in the midst of early debates about evidence-based practice. Usually, the debates about definitions or the discourse in the process vs. specific treatment model debates ignored the key and parallel development of this science that is essential to producing improved client outcomes. Subsequent chapters in this book provide a detailed examination of program implementation.*

References

Barwick, M. (2011). Master's level clinician competencies in child and youth behavioral healthcare. *Emotional & Behavioral Disorders in Youth, 11*(2), 32–39.

Bertram, R. M., Blase, K. A., & Fixsen, D. L. (2015). Improving programs and outcomes: Implementation frameworks and organization change. *Research on Social Work Practice, 25*(4), 477–487.

Bertram, R. M., Charnin, L. A., Kerns, S. E. U., & Long, A. C. (2015). Evidence-based practices in North American MSW curricula. *Research on Social Work Practice, 25*(6), 737-748.

Bertram, R. M., Choi, S. W., & Elsen, M. (2018). Integrating implementation science and evidence-based practice into academic and field curricula. *Journal of Social Work Education,* 1–11.

Bertram, R. M., King, K., Pederson, R., & Nutt, J. (2014). Program implementation: An examination of the interface of curriculum and practice. *Journal of Evidence-Based Social Work, 11,* 193–207.

Bettinger, E. P., & Long, B. T. (2010). Does cheaper mean better? The impact of using adjunct instructors on student outcomes. *The Review of Economics and Statistics, 92*(3), 598–613.

Bruns, E. J., Kerns, S. E. U., Pullmann, M. D., Hensley, S. W., Lutterman, T., & Hoagwood, K. E. (2015). Research, data, and evidence-based treatment use in state behavioral health systems, 2001–2012. *Psychiatric Services, 67*(5), 496–503.

Cannata, E., Marlowe, D.B., Bertram, R. Kerns, S.E.U., Wolfe, S. & Choi, S. (in progress). *A comparison of evidence-based practice in social work and marriage and family therapy master degree programs.*

Chambless, D. L., & Hollon, S. D. (1998). Defining empirically supported therapies. *Journal of Consulting and Clinical Psychology, 66,* 7–18.

Chambless, D. L., & Ollendick, T. H. (2001). Empirically supported psychological interventions: Controversies and evidence. *Annual Review of Psychology, 52,* 685–716.

Commission on Accreditation for Marriage and Family Therapy Education. (2017). *Accreditation standards: Graduate & post-graduate marriage and family therapy training programs,* version 12.0. Alexandria: Author.

Council on Social Work Education. (2015). *Educational policy and accreditation standards.* Alexandria: Author.

Drabick, D. A., & Goldfried, M. R. (2000). Training the scientist–practitioner for the 21st century: Putting the bloom back on the rose. *Journal of Clinical Psychology, 56,* 327–340.

Fixsen, D. L., Blase, K. A., Naoom, S. F., & Wallace, F. (2009). Core implementation components. *Research on Social Work Practice, 19*(5), 531–540.

Fixsen, D. L., Naoom, S. F., Blase, K. A., Friedman, R. M., & Wallace, F. (2005). *Implementation research: A synthesis of the literature.* Tampa: University of South Florida, Louis de la Parte Florida Mental Health Institute, The National Implementation Research Network (FMHI Publication #231).

Frank, G. (1984). The Boulder model: History, rationale, and critique. *Professional Psychology: Research and Practice, 15,* 417–435.

Howard, M. O., McMillen, J. C., & Pollio, D. E. (2003). Teaching evidence-based practice: Toward a new paradigm for social work education. *Journal of Research on Social Work Practice, 13*, 234–259.

Insel, T. (2015, July 14). Post by former NIMH director Thomas Insel: Quality counts [Blog post]. Retrieved from https://www.nimh.nih.gov/about/directors/thomas-insel/blog/2015/quality-counts.shtml.

Institute of Medicine. (2015). *Psychosocial interventions for mental and substance use disorders: A framework for establishing evidence-based standards.* Washington, DC: The National Academies Press.

Kanary, P. J., Bertram, R. M., & Bernstein, D. (2017). The child and family evidence-based practice consortium: Pathways to the future. *Families in Society: The Journal of Contemporary Social Services, 98*(1), 7–8.

Kazdin, A. E., Bass, D., Ayers, W. A., & Rodgers, A. (1990). Empirical and clinical focus of child and adolescent psychotherapy research. *Journal of Consulting and Clinical Psychology, 58*(6), 729–740.

Karam, E. A., & Sprenkle, D. H. (2010). The research-informed clinician: A guide to training the next generation MFT. *Journal of Marital and Family Therapy, 36*(3), 307–319.

Meyer, A. S., Templeton, G. B., Stinson, M. A., & Codone, S. (2016). Teaching research methods to MFT Master's students: A comparison between scientist-practitioner and research-informed approaches. *Contemporary Family Therapy, 38*(3), 295–306.

Oka, M., & Whiting, J. (2013). Bridging the clinician/researcher gap with systemic research: The case for process research, dyadic, and sequential analysis. *Journal of Marital and Family Therapy, 39*(1), 17–27.

Owenz, M., & Hall, S. R. (2011). Bridging the research-practice gap in psychotherapy training: Qualitative analysis of master's students' experiences in a student-led research and practice team. *North American Journal of Psychology, 13*(1).

Parker, E. O., Chang, J., & Thomas, V. (2016). A content analysis of quantitative research in journal of marital and family therapy: A 10-year review. *Journal of Marital and Family Therapy, 42*(1), 3–18.

Parrish, D. E., & Rubin, A. (2012). Social workers' orientations toward the evidence-based practice process: A comparison with psychologists and licensed marriage and family therapists. *Social Work, 57*(3), 201–210.

Proctor, E. K. (2007). Implementing evidence-based practice in social work education: Principles, strategies, and partnerships. *Research on Social Work Practice, 17*(5), 583–591.

Raimy, V. (Ed.). (1950). *Training in clinical psychology.* Prentice-Hall.

Silverman, W. K., & Hinshaw, S. P. (2008). The second special issue on evidence-based psychosocial treatments for children and adolescents: A 10-year update. *Journal of Clinical Child and Adolescent Psychology, 37*, 1–7.

Stith, S. M. (2014). What does this mean for graduate education in marriage and family therapy? commentary on "The divide between 'evidenced–based' approaches and practitioners of traditional theories of family therapy". *Journal of Marital and Family Therapy, 40*(1), 17–19.

Thyer, B. A., & Myers, L. L. (2011). The quest for evidence-based practice: A view from the United States. *Journal of Social Work, 11*, 8–25.

Chapter 6
Establishing Effectiveness: An Innovation Tale

For years, program developers devised innovative practices in university settings that reliably treated a host of emotional and behavioral health problems only to find that when they disseminated the innovative practice into community settings, its effectiveness diminished, and often quite considerably. This is a substantial concern for treatment developers and communities.

Efficacy Trial

For our next allegorical tale, let's examine how innovative practices were proven effective and disseminated before implementation science emerged. Imagine that a researcher developed an innovative practice model for parents experiencing difficulties with the behavior of their children attending kindergarten through elementary school (ages five to twelve). She wrote a grant and received funding for an *efficacy trial* to study the practice within her laboratory at the university. Graduate students served as the primary practitioners. They received intensive training and individualized coaching from the researcher. Sessions with parents and their identified child were videotaped. The researcher reviewed videotapes with the graduate student practitioners in a two-hour group supervision every week.

Families participating in the *efficacy trial* were recruited from communities near the university through invitations available at parent–teacher conferences, as well as by posting invitations at grocery stores, healthcare clinics, and in local papers. Treatment was provided at no charge to the families, but they were expected to have transportation to participate in all sessions and to pay for campus parking.

This researcher was very diligent and met all of her recruitment and treatment goals and timelines. The *efficacy trial* was highly successful. Over 80% of the families experienced clinically significant improvements in their child's behavior.

© Springer Nature Switzerland AG 2019
R. Bertram and S. Kerns, *Selecting and Implementing Evidence-Based Practice*,
https://doi.org/10.1007/978-3-030-11325-4_6

However, five years passed between the initial grant award and the analysis and submission of the *efficacy trial* results for publication. This included nearly a year of clinical trial preparation that included completing Human Subjects Institutional Review Board (IRB) protocols, hiring and training graduate student practitioners, and preparing the treatment rooms with video and audio equipment, etc. Two years were spent recruiting and enrolling parents and delivering the innovative practice model. After the last client completed treatment, there was one year of follow-up activities to track sustainability of improvements in the children's behaviors, and an additional year to completely analyze, write, and submit results to a journal where peer-review could take another six months to a year before the study was finally published.

Effectiveness Trial

Based on these impressive results, the researcher received her next grant to conduct an *effectiveness trial* of the intervention. This support allowed her to move the now innovative, promising practice from the research clinic to the local community where she had a good working relationship with administrators and supervisors at a behavioral healthcare center. They committed their organization to serve as the location for the *effectiveness trial*.

With the researcher, they developed a staff training and client recruitment plan. In this study, graduate students would not serve as practitioners. Instead, in three days of training, the behavioral healthcare clinicians were taught essential elements and activities of the innovative promising practice model. They received weekly individual telephone consultation from the researcher during the time period their clients participated in the study. Sessions with parents and their identified child were videotaped, so the researcher could assess fidelity. However, due to the complexities of coordinating so many schedules, she did not review videotapes with the clinicians.

Unlike the *efficacy trial*, this was a randomized controlled study. Families were recruited by staff and by placing invitations to participate throughout the busy behavioral healthcare center. Like the previous study, families had to transport themselves, this time to the behavioral healthcare center, but there was ample free parking. Unlike that *efficacy trial*, whether assigned to the experimental group or to the control group, families paid for treatment.

This two-year *effectiveness trial* initially suffered from low client recruitment. The study's research design required fifty families to be enrolled to participate in the experimental group receiving the innovative promising practice. Fifty others would comprise the control group receiving usual clinic interventions for such child behavior problems. However, at the end of the first year, only 20 families enrolled in the study and only 17 of these completed all treatment sessions. Because it seemed that there would not be sufficient families available, the researcher convinced another behavioral healthcare center in an adjacent community to participate. She had to then train those clinicians and work with the center to recruit clients. A few more families entered the study, but at the end of the second year of enrollment, she still only had 35 families who had enrolled and completed all treatment sessions.

The researcher requested and received a no-cost extension from her funder. Finally, after one more year of recruiting, the study was able to complete treatment with 50 enrolled families. All participating families were recruited from the community behavioral healthcare agencies during their intake process or they were current clients. Similar to the university-based *efficacy trial*, families were expected to have transportation to participate in the treatment sessions. However, for this *effectiveness trial*, families also had to have insurance so the agencies could bill for clinician time and efforts. This *effectiveness trial* was successful, with 75% of families experiencing clinically significant improvements in their child's behavior.

This *effectiveness trial* took six years to complete and publish. This included a year of preparation to secure agreements with the initial behavioral healthcare center and to complete IRB protocols, as well as to train clinicians, and prepare rooms with video and audio equipment, etc. Due to the low initial enrollment and engagement of an additional behavioral healthcare center, it took three years before enough families participated in all sessions of the innovative promising practice model. As in the *efficacy trial*, there was one year of follow-up activities to track sustainability of improvements in the children's behaviors, and an additional year to completely analyze, write, and submit results to a journal that could take another six months to a year before the study was published.

Though she was very proud of results from the randomized controlled *effectiveness trial* study, the researcher had concern that the now **evidence-based practice model** might not be generalizable for diverse families. When she looked at the families who participated in the two studies, most were Euro-American (75%) and had insurance and transportation supported by moderate incomes. There was some improvement in income and cultural diversity in the *effectiveness trial* because approximately 50% of the families had Medicaid insurance. Nevertheless, communities served by the two behavioral healthcare centers were not racially diverse. Most concerning to this researcher, only 3% of her sample were linguistically diverse. This was not enough of her sample to analyze results separately for different client characteristics, but anecdotally it seemed there were additional barriers to participation and treatment challenges for those families where English was not the primary language spoken.

Transportability or Dissemination Study

Next, the researcher addressed how this now **evidence-based practice model** would translate in both language and activities for parents with limited English proficiency. She sought colleagues in other parts of the country to recruit a more diverse sample. After a year of discussions and leveraging her professional network, she partnered with a research group in a region where 72% of families speak Spanish. Together they wrote a successful grant to fund replicating the now **evidence-based practice model** with this population of families. Similar to the prior grants, practitioners were recruited from the local behavioral healthcare center and preference was given to those with several years of post-graduate experience who could provide the evidence-based practice model in Spanish. During the planning year, all materials had to be translated and back translated to ensure that the practice model elements and activities were clear in both English and Spanish.

The researchers also conducted focus groups with local community members to review the practice model and determine if there were any elements or activities that could be interpreted differently due to language and cultural considerations. A few minor changes resulted from this process, but the key elements and activities and how they contributed to improved outcomes (theory of change) remained largely the same. An additional step was taken to identify recruitment strategies that would increase the likelihood families would enroll in the study, including hiring a cultural liaison.

These efforts were very successful, and within two years, there were sufficient families enrolled in the randomized controlled *dissemination study* (sometimes called a *transportability trial*). This study also took approximately 5 years to complete client recruitment, clinician training and consultation, as well as follow-up activities and analysis. Results were good, with 72% of families experiencing clinically significant improvements in child behavior. Additionally, the more experienced Spanish-speaking community-based practitioners delivered the adapted evidence-based model with moderate to high levels of treatment fidelity and few challenges to clinic-based implementation.

Given the success of the efficacy, effectiveness, and transportability studies, the practice model had moved from an innovation to a promising practice to an evidence-based practice proven effective with diverse populations and became eligible for higher ratings in various practice registries (see Chap. 3 and the appendix at the conclusion of this book for a description of some registries). After 17 years, this researcher was finally confident to begin to transport the evidence-based practice to other communities and service settings in other parts of the country. Not surprisingly, prior to the emergence of implementation science, seventeen years was the average length of time it takes for interventions to proceed from early efficacy trials to effectiveness trials and ultimately be ready for dissemination and transport to other settings (Balas & Boren, 2000).

However, note that the initial researcher's focus was on treatment development, *not* on embedding and implementing the evidence-based practice in an organization or service. This example highlights a very typical pathway for treatment development that often leaves important questions that could inform implementation unanswered. For example, none of the researchers' studies addressed how fidelity could be assessed by non-research staff. How could agency supervisors or specialists coach practitioners to greater competence and confidence in delivering this evidence-based practice? None of the studies examined staff selection and whether there was an optimal professional or experiential background for practitioners. None of the studies examined transportability to other settings. Could the *evidence-based practice model* be delivered effectively, with fidelity, as an in-home service or in a school or church setting? With the emergence of implementation science, these sorts of questions can now be actively considered and tested as part of the process of disseminating and transporting innovative evidence-based practices to other settings or contexts.

Hybrid Studies

This established process that establishes a sound evidence base for a new program or practice slows its eventual delivery in community settings. Even under ideal conditions, it can take many years to establish the requisite evidence in efficacy, effectiveness, and dissemination or transportability studies. One potential strategy for addressing this challenge is the development of hybrid studies that simultaneously test effectiveness and implementation (Bernet, Willens, & Bauer, 2012). There are three primary types of hybrid studies: (1) Type I: Rigorous testing of the effectiveness of the intervention while collecting critical implementation-related information; (2) Type II: Rigorous testing of the effectiveness of the intervention and rigorous testing of the implementation method; and (3) Type III: Testing the implementation method while collecting client outcome data.

Summary

The process of successfully completing efficacy trials, then effectiveness trials, followed by dissemination or transportability studies establishes a sound evidence base for a new program or practice. However, it takes time and slows its eventual delivery to clients in community settings. Hybrid studies can speed this process, but all studies of programs or practices must eventually address their implementation in community settings.

References

Balas, E. A., & Boren, S. A. (2000). Managing clinical knowledge for health care improvement. *Yearbook of Medical Informatics 2000: Patient-Centered Systems,* (1), 65–70.

Bernet, A. C., Willens, D. E., & Bauer, M. S. (2012). Effectiveness-implementation hybrid designs: Implications for quality improvement science. *Implementation Science, 8*(Suppl 1), S2.

Chapter 7
An Explorer's Guide
to Evidence-Based Practice

Just as the explorer's guide to the universe walks readers through the history of how knowledge about the evolution of discoveries of the universe (Gregersen, 2010), in this chapter we take readers on a journey through the generation of evidence that establishes a practice model as evidence-based, research-based, or a promising practice. We will examine and discuss:

- Early efforts to define practice components and move treatments from efficacy to effectiveness trials;
- The need to develop fidelity measures—first to establish internal validity for treatment studies and later to ensure adequate transport within real-world settings; and
- Efforts to unpack common practice elements and mechanisms of change, to help inform treatment adaptations for specific populations.

Additionally, we discuss the most efficacious approaches to treatment of common concerns, such as anxiety, depression, traumatic stress, and child behavior problems. Finally, in this chapter we present an example of how a strategically selected set of evidence-based, research-based, and promising practice models could be installed within a system of care to address a majority of community, family and individual concerns. However, the most effective treatment models are frequently not available in many communities, and even when available, the quality and extent to which they are provided with fidelity is often unknown.

This phenomenon is called the "science-to-practice gap," or even more bluntly, the "quality chasm." In previous chapters, we identified how academic professional degree programs contribute to this gap between what we know works and what we actually do. There are also organizational factors that maintain this gap and contribute to why proven practice models experience diminished effectiveness when delivered in communities. In this chapter, we begin to explore multiple organizational factors that contribute to the science-to-practice gap in evidence-based practice, as well as the means to address them.

© Springer Nature Switzerland AG 2019
R. Bertram and S. Kerns, *Selecting and Implementing Evidence-Based Practice*,
https://doi.org/10.1007/978-3-030-11325-4_7

The Process of Proving Effectiveness

In Chap. 3, we identified how definitions for *evidence-based practice models* and for a *process of evidence-based practice* emerged from the field of medicine. This biomedical origin is also the basis for the development of behavioral treatment models.

In medicine, early-stage clinical trials are conducted, typically, in laboratory settings and often with non-human animals. If these trials are successful, then highly controlled experimental trials are conducted with a select group of patients who are willing to take risks with experimental drugs or procedures. Then, if these trials seem successful and the benefits outweigh possible adverse side effects, a larger clinical study occurs. Through this careful, scientific process, the drugs or procedures become available for the general population with similar medical concerns. This process can take three to five years under ideal conditions.

Historically, development of behavioral health treatment models follows a similar pattern. First, the innovative practice is tested with a very well-defined client population. For example, a particular client age group may be identified, and from this group, only those with the specific behavior of concern are selected as study subjects. If a person displays multiple behaviors of concern (called "comorbidity"), they are excluded from the study. Usually, at this early stage there are limitations on whether they can be taking psychotropic medications and, if they are permitted, the dose must remain stable across the clinical trial. In essence, researchers attempt to completely isolate the specific problem that needs to be impacted and tightly control everything else. This is called an *efficacy trial*.

This process is important to establish internal validity, the assurance that you are, in fact, studying what you intend to study and not accidentally studying something else. For example, if you are studying an innovative treatment for social anxiety, you must ensure that your sample subjects indeed experience social anxiety, with no other disorders present, such as an obsessive-compulsive disorder that could compromise testing the innovative treatment for social anxiety. Under these highly controlled conditions, the intervention is then tested. Typically, the research team either personally delivers or closely monitors and supervises practitioners who deliver the innovative treatment. This often occurs in university-based clinics or hospitals. If the innovative treatment has its desired outcome, then researchers conduct *effectiveness trials*.

Effectiveness trials are designed to test treatment effects under more "real-world" conditions. This means that there is more flexibility for clients to display characteristics more similar to the general population. This could include other behaviors of concern (comorbid) and/or concerns that are managed with psychotropic medications. There still may be some exclusionary criteria, but in general and by design, *effectiveness trials* are meant to be more inclusive than the *efficacy trials*. The other main difference is that *effectiveness trials* test the innovative treatment in more traditional mental health treatment settings or in schools. Thus, during this phase of testing, the innovative treatment may be delivered by community-based practitioners. There may still be substantial technical assistance provided by the researchers to ensure that the innovative treatment model is delivered as intended. However, because it is delivered by practitioners in community-based settings, *effectiveness trials* also ensure that the innovative treatment can be replicated. This is called external validity. *Effectiveness trials* demonstrate that the innovative treatment model achieves robust outcomes in more generalizable settings.

As you can see, there is often a balancing act or tension between internal and external validity. Researchers must make careful decisions about when to sacrifice internal validity for the sake of external validity, and vice versa. For example, a study may want to ensure internal validity by limiting the age of clients accepted for the study. Researchers may choose to include only 9–10-year-old children in the study to control for factors such as brain/cognitive development. This age restriction would increase the internal validity of the study because it would rule out or substantially limit possible variables such as brain development and the impact of onset of puberty. However, it is unlikely that a program with such a restricted age would be appealing to community-based providers who are charged with serving a large age range of children and adolescents. Therefore, another option would be to tip the balance to have greater external validity by expanding the age range of study subjects, say from 8 to 15. In this case, researchers would statistically control for age and other factors that might impact outcomes. Depending on what outcomes are associated with the intervention, they might control for prior history of the behavioral concern, prior involvement in the justice or special education system, or other variables that have strong correlation with the outcome (i.e., could predict the outcome absent of the intervention) to strengthen the study.

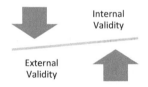

Another example of this tension between internal and external validity would be a study that uses a very stringent method of quality assurance to ensure internal validity. This could mean that every treatment session is taped and reviewed with the practitioner prior to the next session. In this way, adherence to model elements and activities (fidelity) is closely monitored and tracked. Researchers in this case would be very confident about exactly what intervention the client received. However, researchers concerned with external validity may design an approach to its implementation that more closely mimics what is practical in community-based settings. They may sacrifice the precision of the first method for a more pragmatic approach that is potentially more generalizable to a variety of settings by having practitioners self-report treatment elements.

Every study's research team may make different decisions about addressing internal and external validity, so it is important to closely and critically examine design and methods sections of articles (see Chap. 3 for a brief discussion of selecting and critically examining publications) so you can determine how relevant a practice may be for a particular population or setting. Astute readers may also recall that in Chap. 3, this scientific process was basis for some early criticisms and resistance to evidence-based practice.

Even well-written grants often have challenges with participant recruitment and maintaining requisite human subject protection approvals. They often experience protracted peer-review publication timelines of a year or more. The careful process of moving from establishing efficacy to effectiveness to eventual dissemination is a long one. However, most innovative practice models are not designed with broad-scale implementation and dissemination in mind. Despite efficacy and effectiveness trials, there may be features of the innovative treatment model that are not feasible in many community settings.

For example, there is a parenting intervention that was tested as an approach for addressing oppositional behaviors in children between the ages of three and eight. It was designed to be delivered in 90-min sessions twice per week, for approximately three months. One or both parents along with the identified child were required to be present. In special sessions, and only after skill mastery, parents could later bring other children in the home who were also within the study's proscribed age range.

This intervention was evaluated and was highly effective in helping parents to successfully manage oppositional behavior in their children. However, this innovative treatment model had several features that made it difficult to transport into community settings. Few clinics are prepared for families to come multiple times per week, and insurance reimbursement guidelines might limit the number of sessions. In addition to clinics not having the time slots and related space available, the number of sessions per week was also burdensome for families because transportation and childcare can pose substantial practical challenges to their participation in treatment. Because ninety-minute sessions are unusual in many community-based clinics, this requirement could present a financial disincentive for agencies that then may need to fill an extra thirty-minute billable service slot. Because this innovative treatment model required parents to initially only bring the "identified child," it created a clear burden for childcare, especially if there was an infant in the family. Finally and further related to external validity, when parents return home, the distractions of the other children can produce substantial challenges to consistent application of abilities developed in the clinic. Planning for such distractions in a clinic session can be helpful, but having opportunity to practice managing them directly is even better.

So, what did the innovative treatment developers do? They offered some suggestions for adapting the intervention to better fit a more typical clinical context, including delivering the intervention in hour-long sessions once per week, and accommodating the presence of other children if necessary. Will these changes impact treatment effectiveness? This is currently being tested. However, if these structural changes were considered earlier, they could have been tested during the effectiveness (or even efficacy) trials and we would have the answer to this critical question. If considered early in the process of model development, researchers can ensure that innovative treatments will not need to be retrofitted to be able to be scaled and disseminated successfully into community settings.

The Importance of Treatment Fidelity

Documenting that an innovative practice was delivered as intended is an essential step in the process of evaluating its outcomes. When improved outcomes are not achieved, there are two possible explanations: (1) the innovative practice is not effective or (2) it was not delivered with fidelity. As the testing of an innovative practice moves from more highly controlled university-based settings and *efficacy trials* into community-based settings and *effectiveness trials*, evaluating treatment fidelity becomes critical to support its transportability to other settings.

In fact, some studies show that when evidence-based treatment models are not delivered as intended, there can actually be iatrogenic effects (create more harm than good). In such cases, clients are better off not receiving the treatment at all than receiving a poorly delivered one. An intriguing study conducted by Hogue et al. (2008) examined whether two different treatments (Cognitive Behavioral Therapy (CBT) or Multidimensional Family Therapy (MDFT) had any effect on adolescent substance use. This study shows the complicated nature of the relationship between treatment fidelity and outcomes. For marijuana use, greater therapist adherence (fidelity) was related to less marijuana use for the CBT treatment group but not the MDFT group. In both treatment groups, greater therapist adherence (fidelity) was related to reductions in parent-reported ratings of externalizing symptoms (i.e., behavior problems such as conduct problems and attention-deficit hyperactivity disorder). A fascinating relationship was found between adherence and outcomes for internalizing symptoms (i.e., mood-related problems such as anxiety and depression). Those with moderate adherence had the clients with the lowest internalizing symptoms. Greater symptoms were found for those with both low and high adherence. What do we take from this study? It is important to "stick to the program" but not so rigidly that individual needs are compromised. Some authors have provided guidelines for considering flexibility within fidelity (e.g., Forehand, Dorsey, Jones, Long, & McMahon, 2010; Mazzucchelli & Sanders, 2010).

In 2011, Thomas Sexton and Charles Turner published a study on Functional Family Therapy (Sexton & Turner, 2011). *In this study, they found that the youth who had therapists with high levels of adherence to the treatment model had significantly positive and highly impactful clinical outcomes compared to those youth in the control condition.*

However, the youth who had the therapists with lower adherence to the treatment model had significantly worse outcomes compared to the control condition. In this case, the youth with poorly adherent therapists were worse off.

Treatment fidelity measurement challenges. Several challenges have occurred when treatment developers attempted to use the same treatment fidelity assessment strategies used in efficacy or effectiveness trials when they transport the innovative treatment into community settings. So-called gold standard treatment fidelity assessment typically includes either live observation or videotaped review of sessions, followed by intensive coaching feedback (Sholomaskas et al., 2005). Sometimes ongoing consultation calls are required. Led by a model developer or expert in the innovative evidence-based practice, these are typically hour-long calls that occur once per week, every other week, or monthly. Some treatment developers require ongoing consultation for the entire duration of the time a practitioner is delivering the intervention. Multisystemic Therapy uses this approach. Others require time-limited consultation (e.g., six months or a year). Trauma-Focused Cognitive Behavioral Therapy (TF-CBT) typically requires six months of consultation with a treatment expert. A few require competency-based consultation in which practitioners receive consultation until they demonstrate proficiency in the model. Examples of these interventions include Solution-Based Casework, Functional Family Therapy, and Parent–Child Interaction Therapy.

However, requiring this type of consultation for fidelity assessment is limiting. There are a finite number of people capable of providing expert feedback and this limits the extent of model dissemination that can be supported. Additionally, practitioner time in these activities is not minimal. Each hour they must spend in specialized supervision or consultation activities limits the time they are able to provide billable services. Finally, securing buy-in from practitioners about the relevance and importance of fidelity monitoring and supports can be difficult. Graduate curricula rarely address the necessity or processes for ensuring fidelity, nor how to take advantage of these competences and confidence enhancing supports. Despite these challenges, it is critical to ensure that evidence-based treatments are delivered as intended. It is likewise important for treatment developers to consider strategies that support practical assessments of treatment fidelity in community settings.

Sonja Schoenwald authored "It's a Bird, It's a Plane, It's … Fidelity Measurement in the Real World" (Schoenwald, 2011). In this commentary, she challenges the field to establish fidelity tools that are feasible and pragmatic within practice settings. Fidelity is no longer the domain of researchers seeking to ensure that study participants received the intervention as intended. Now, fidelity assessments are sometimes used to assess program quality and can have impacts on fiscal supports and client referrals.

An emerging use of fidelity assessment is to incorporate fidelity data into supervision protocols. For example, Shannon Dorsey and colleagues are examining a strategy of having supervisors use symptom and fidelity monitoring as a primary strategy to enhance supervision. They are testing the impact of this alone and are combining this with supervising and guiding clinician behavioral rehearsal (Dorsey et al., 2013).

Effective Treatment Models

In the past three decades, hundreds of treatment studies identified effective practices that address a range of emotional and behavioral disorders. Among the most common are treatments for anxiety, depression, attention-deficit hyperactivity disorder (ADHD), traumatic stress, conduct disorders and substance use disorders. These include Parent–Child Interaction Therapy (for conduct problems), Dialectical Behavior Therapy (for internalizing symptoms including suicide risk and borderline personality disorder), Trauma-Focused Cognitive Behavioral Therapy (for symptoms of traumatic stress), Multisystemic Therapy (for conduct problems and substance use disorders) and so many more. Each model identifies specific populations and settings for which they are effective. Each may have age or symptom severity qualifications and service locations (e.g., home-based, office-based, school-based). They may also identify structural parameters such as if it is a family, group, or individual treatment, as well as the frequency and intensity of sessions, session requirements, etc. The following is a very brief review of the most effective treatments for the most common emotional and behavioral problems in children and youth. Readers can search for others through Web-based registries highlighted in the Appendix at the end of this book.

Treatment of anxiety. The underlying principle in anxiety treatment is that anxiety is maintained by avoidance. For example, if you are afraid of spiders, every time you see a spider, you run away. By running away, you are able to recover from your anxiety response. This reinforces the behavior of avoiding spiders. Therefore, the only way to treat anxiety is to be exposed to that which is causing the anxiety. You would never recover from your fear of spiders if you arranged your life so you would never encounter a spider. Fear of crowds, airplanes, dogs, the dark, separation from a parent, etc., is often maintained by avoidance. If these fears result in functional impacts such as preventing someone from going to school, socializing with friends, leaving their house, or otherwise participating in their life, anxiety-related symptoms must be effectively and efficiently addressed.

There are different ways to approach treatment of anxiety disorders. Typically, in children from age 7 or 8 through 17, it is recommended that clinicians use a procedure called gradual exposure (Kendall, Crawford, Kagan, Furr, & Podell, 2003). Children collaborate with their practitioner to build a "fear ladder" that contains different scenarios of varying levels of anxiety intensity. Given the spider example above, a practitioner might use lower levels of intensity such as viewing pictures of a spider, watching video of a moving spider, seeing a stuffed animal spider, and then holding the stuffed animal spider. Clinicians applying moderate levels of gradual exposure intensity could show the child a dead spider in a box, or remove the dead spider for viewing outside the box or encourage the child to observe a live spider in a box. The highest levels of gradual exposure anxiety would likely be caused by seeing a live spider out of a box and finally holding a live spider. Of course, there is individual variability in subjective experiences of anxiety, so these anxiety levels may be different for different people. With gradual exposure, practitioners work with the client to learn effective coping and calming techniques and then to apply these techniques to tolerate each level of exposure, eventually working up to their most feared scenario. There are nuances to this approach and it should only be undertaken by someone with training and supervision in the anxiety protocols for the many practice models that apply it. Caution-training, and supervision are essential because a "failed" exposure, one in which the client is able to escape from the feared situation before their anxiety is brought under control, can make the situation worse and increase the likelihood that the client will not return to get help with their fear.

Other approaches for the treatment of anxiety include flooding and imaginal exposure, both of which are typically more appropriate for adults. Flooding is when a client confronts whatever their primary fear is and they are required to remain in the situation until their anxiety abates. Imaginal exposure is when there is never an actual exposure. Rather the client is directed to imagine various scenarios in which they might encounter their fear. However, neither of these approaches are typically the first choice for treatment of children, especially those under 13 or 14 years of age. Flooding can be experienced as highly stressful and, while adults can be explained the treatment procedures and rationale, children may not have as much cognitive agency over their therapeutic experience. Imaginal exposure is a challenge because of cognitive development-related complications.

Another popular evidence-based treatment for children experiencing anxiety between the ages of 7 and 13 is "Coping Cat." Developed by Phil Kendall and colleagues (Kendall, 2006), Coping Cat teaches children to identify anxiety in their brain and body and helps them to think through how to understand their thoughts and feelings in situations when they are feeling anxious. They then learn effective coping strategies and are taught to give themselves positive reinforcement when they effectively use their skills. Treatment is delivered in weekly sessions for approximately 16 weeks. While the treatment is delivered predominately with the youth, parents are involved directly in several sessions. The primary outcome of this program is reductions in youth anxiety. Across numerous research studies, approximately 20–25% of the treatment sample was of an ethnicity other than white.

Treatment of traumatic stress symptoms. Some common reactions to exposure to trauma include experiencing bad memories, avoiding places, people, or other reminders of the traumatic event, having the traumatic event unexpectedly pop into thoughts, experiencing disrupted sleep or nightmares, overwhelming feelings of numbness or hopelessness, difficulty concentrating and being overly alert (hypervigilant). When these symptoms last for a long time and interfere with daily functioning, it may be diagnosed as post-traumatic stress disorder (PTSD). The most effective treatments for PTSD are cognitive behavioral approaches that work with the client to differentiate the traumatic memory from otherwise safe situations that cause distress (e.g., trauma triggers).

While there are many treatments for PTSD, only a few have strong evidence for effectiveness. A terrific resource for PTSD treatment approaches for both children and adults is Foa, Keane, Friedman, and Cohen (2008) book: *Effective treatments for PTSD: Practice guidelines from the International Society for Traumatic Stress Studies*. For children, individually focused Cognitive Behavioral Therapy (CBT) with parent involvement, individually focused CBT, and group CBT have the best evidence (Dorsey et al., 2017).

This includes Trauma-Focused Cognitive Behavioral Therapy (TF-CBT; Cohen, Mannarino, & Deblinger, 2006), one of the most extensively researched interventions for traumatic stress. This *evidence-based treatment model* follows a protocol described through the acronym: PRACTICE. The P stands for psychoeducation and parenting skills; R stands for relaxation; A stands for affect identification and modulation; C stands for cognitive coping; T stands for the trauma narrative; I stands for in vivo desensitization; C stands for preparing for a conjoint session between the child and a caregiver; and E stands for establishing safety. With the exception of establishing safety, which can be instituted at any point needed throughout treatment, by and large the practitioner goes through each of step in that order with the client. Treatment typically lasts 8–16 sessions but varies depending on client needs. Other treatment models for children with emerging evidence include Trauma Systems Therapy (Saxe, Ellis, & Kaplow, 2007) and Child–Parent Psychotherapy (Lieberman, Van Horn, & Ippen 2005).

For adults, Prolonged Exposure Therapy may be a treatment of choice (Foa et al., 2005). Clients are taught to face their fears and memories through individual treatment sessions. Clients learn to retell their traumatic story and process the thoughts and feelings associated with the memory. Therapists will work with a client to develop a "fear hierarchy" of reminders or triggers that are causing distress and help the client to learn to approach those otherwise safe people, situations, or memories.

Treatment of depression. Cognitive behavioral approaches are typically the most effective for treatment of depression in children, adolescents, and adults. Teaching clients about the connection between thoughts, feelings, and behaviors is an important component of treatment. Behavioral activation includes scheduling activities that a client may be avoiding because of their depression. This could include going for walks, answering the phone, exercising, participating in errands, and other common day-to-day activities. Cognitive strategies may include identifying and challenging unhelpful or automatic thoughts (e.g., "nobody loves me"; or, "he did that on purpose just to irritate me!").

Relaxation techniques are often part of depression treatment. These can include techniques such as purposeful breathing, progressive muscle relaxation, and imaginal relaxation. For purposeful breathing, clients are taught how to use their breath to relax. In its most simple form, practitioners coach clients to attend to their breath for a few minutes while focusing on deep, diaphragmatic breathing (filling up your belly like a balloon when you breathe in). In a more advanced breathing technique, the client is coached to use their fingers to facilitate alternate breathing. First the client closes their left nostril, and inhales through the right nostril. They then open their left nostril, close the right one, and exhale through their left nostril. Then they inhale through the left, and exhale through the right. Then they inhale through the right nostril, and exhale through the left. Clients are taught to alternate this pattern for about 10 rounds (one round begins and ends on the right side). A word of caution if any of you are trying this at home—be sure you can breathe freely through both nostrils. This technique does not work well if you have a cold!

Progressive muscle relaxation is typically a guided practice in which the client is taught to tighten and release a variety of large muscles through their body. There are some fabulous apps that help to provide guidance. Because individual preference is paramount for continued use, we recommend trying out different apps or resources to ensure finding one that works.

Imaginal relaxation is conducted when a client is guided to think of a relaxing place. Often, they are guided through imaging each of their senses. For example, if a client is thinking about being on the beach, they would be encouraged to think about how the sand feels on their feet, the breeze in their hair and on their cheeks, the salty fresh smell, the sound of the seagulls overhead, and the warmth of the sun.

For children, one of the more effective treatments for treatment of depression is called Primary and Secondary Control Enhancement Training (PASCET). This treatment was developed by Weisz et al. (2005). It was developed for children between the ages of 8–15 who have symptoms of depression. Over the course of approximately 10–17 individual sessions, children are taught to differentiate between events in which they have control (primary) and those situations in which they do not have control. For primary control, they are taught to problem solve their situation and develop mastery over the situation. For situations when they do not have control, they are taught coping strategies and other ways to adjust to the situation (thus, creating secondary control). Another effective intervention is called Interpersonal Treatment for Adolescents (ITP-A; Mufson & Moreau, 1999). This 12-week treatment for adolescent depression combines psychoeducation and skill building. Psychoeducation includes teaching the youth about depression, how it impacts their life, and how treatment works. Adolescents work on communication and interpersonal effectiveness. They also learn problem-solving strategies. Treatment is conducted first in a clinic setting and youth then work to apply the skills to their own lives.

Treatment of conduct problems. The underlying theory-based principle in treatment of conduct problems is that behaviors have a function that is maintained by factors in the environment. Behavioral theories suggest that most behavior can be understood by examining "antecedents" and "consequences." For example, if a youth, let's call him Jack, is yelling at his parents because he wants to go to a party, the function of that behavior is to get something that he wants. The antecedent (i.e., what happened right before the problem behavior) may have been how his parents initially said "no" or how they did not respond to his desire to go to the party. If the parents give in and let him go to the party, then the consequence is that he gets to go to the party and his yelling behavior is reinforced. He is likely to try yelling at them again the next time he wants something. It would be difficult for a practitioner to get very far trying to talk him out of his behavior, especially if he experiences the yelling as effective in getting what he wants.

In this way, most behavior develops because it solves a problem. The child who nags incessantly for a cookie at the grocery store experiences their problem to be solved when their parent gives in and buys one for him. When a teen feels their parents do not care about them and runs away, how the parents convey concern about the runaway may actually reinforce that behavior (therefore, they really do care). A spouse who consistently misses items on the grocery list may be reinforced when the exasperated other spouse takes over the chore (any resemblance to real life events in this example is purely accidental). Back to Jack, the most effective approach to extinguish the boy's yelling is to work with the parents in how they listen to his initial request or how they say no, as well as to not reinforce the problematic behavior by letting him get his way when he is yelling. Instead, they learn to listen and to reinforce skillful behavior such as the boy asking nicely and making responsible choices.

There are many strategies that work to influence antecedents and others that are designed to influence consequences. For younger children (3–8 years), Parent–Child Interaction Therapy (Funderburk & Eyberg, 2011), the Incredible Years (Webster-Stratton & Reid, 2003), the Triple P-Positive Parenting Program (Sanders, 1999), and Helping the Noncompliant Child (McMahon & Forehand, 2005) are all well researched and effective. Interestingly, most of these programs are either "Hanf-based" or "Hanf-inspired" interventions. Constance Hanf was a practitioner at the Oregon Health Sciences University (OHSU) in Portland, OR and developed her model from the mid-1960s through early 1970s (her influence is described in detail in Reitman & McMahon, 2013). While she herself was not a researcher or widely published author, many of our modern-day behavioral parenting experts were trained by her while on their clinical internships. They went on to develop these interventions and rigorously test them. Hanf was ingenious in her technique—once researched her intervention was highly effective. Now, many families have benefited from her wisdom about how to improve child behavior through participating in the above-mentioned interventions.

While there are some differences between the models, they all share a fundamental premise. In order to address child behavior, one must first improve the parent–child relationship and focus on the desirable behaviors you want to see more of. This is done through one-on-one time, praise, paying attention and reflecting positive child behavior, and being clear in giving instructions. Once the relationship is enhanced and positive behaviors are increased, then strategies such as the compliance routine (this includes giving instructions and if a child does not comply, then providing a consequence such as time out or removing a desired activity), planned ignoring (paying no attention to irritating, attention-seeking behaviors), and having standing rules such as no physical aggression. Standing rules have clear consequences for breaking them, such as immediate time out or loss of privileges. Each of the models has different ways to teach parents these skills. PCIT uses a one-way mirror and a bug-in-the-ear to provide real-time coaching. HNC uses in-room coaching between a parent and their child. Both PCIT and HNC are competency-based models. Each has two phases and a parent moves through the program once they demonstrate competency in each area. Triple P has more of a curriculum-based approach, with some live coaching built into the middle of the treatment.

For older youth (12–17), interventions typically are more intensive and involve other systems besides the family (e.g., school, coaches) to support effective behaviors and often include strategies to address substance use or abuse. Examples of such programs are Multisystemic Therapy (Henggeler, Schoenwald, Borduin, Rowland, & Cunningham, 2009) and Functional Family Therapy (Alexander et al., 1998). Multisystemic Therapy (MST) is typically delivered in the family home. It engages the youth, parents/caregivers, and other important people in the youth's life as appropriate. MST is highly individualized for each family. For MST fidelity, individualized family assessment and intervention is guided by nine principles reflecting the model's ecological systems theory base. After a comprehensive assessment of the strengths and struggles of the youth, family, school, peer, and community settings, treatment goals are developed. Primary contributors to the behavior of concern are identified. Working with the family those factors most impacting the problem behavior are targeted for transformation by changing patterns of interaction between the parent, youth, school and others. Guidance from a supervisor and a consultant to the supervisor ensures that assessment and interventions are sustainable and aligned with MST principles. While this is an oversimplified description of MST, it and the example in Chap. 2 demonstrate how treatment is individualized within tested principles. Again, we refer readers to registries discussed in Chap. 3 or in the Appendix at the conclusion of this book for more details about the programs mentioned above.

Common Practice Elements

Briefly discussed in Chap. 3's review of definitions and debates, an interesting and important development in the past several years has been articulation of a *common practice elements approach* toward treatment. Through meta-analyses of empirical literature, there are a number of similar elements or activities across evidence-based practices that appear to be uniquely associated with improved outcomes (e.g., Chorpita, Daleiden, & Weisz, 2005; Kaminski, Valle, Filene, & Boyle, 2008). In these studies, elements or activities that are common across multiple studies are extracted and evaluated. Those that seem to be most closely associated with treatment outcomes are considered "common elements." For example, a common treatment element for anxiety is exposure. Nearly all evidence-based treatments for anxiety contain protocols for exposure, which is described earlier in this chapter. Another example of a common element for treatment of conduct problems in children is specific praise. All evidence-based interventions contain instructions for parents to use specific praise statements (e.g., "I really like how closely you are reading this chapter") to increase desirable behaviors.

Another benefit from *a common elements approach* is that, especially in community mental health settings, clients present with a range of different behavioral health concerns. These concerns may span multiple diagnostic categories of disorder. It may be difficult, if not impossible, for most practitioners to learn a large number of different evidence-based approaches. This may be due to limitations in academic curricula (see Chap. 3). The practitioner's employer may not be able to afford the costs of training and coaching staff in a variety of evidence-based practices. From a practical standpoint, learning and differentiating multiple evidence-based practice model protocols can be challenging.

When clients present with a range of different behavioral health concerns spanning multiple diagnostic categories, practitioners may borrow a little bit here and a little bit there from different practice model protocols. This can compromise fidelity to each model. Further, effective delivery with fidelity of evidence-based practices requires organizational adjustments. Case documentation may need to be aligned to include workbooks or worksheets, forms supporting the appropriate assessment, etc. Props or other materials may be necessary in psychoeducational approaches. Managing and recalling details of multiple practice protocols requires organization and attention and at times may seem overwhelming.

From a financial standpoint, training, coaching and sustaining multiple evidence-based practice models can be expensive. In addition to costs for training and ongoing support, lost revenue during training and coaching and temporary reductions in practitioners' productivity impact the organization's revenue balance sheet. This and concern about staff turnover may limit agency appetite to adopt multiple proven practices. Finally, access to training and support for proven practice is more difficult outside urban areas. For these reasons, common practice elements, or modularized treatment approaches, may be more attractive.

There are emerging models that incorporate *common elements approaches*, these include "Modular Approach to Therapy for Children with Anxiety, Depression, Trauma, or Conduct Problems" (MATCH-ADTC) developed by Chorpita and Weisz (2009) and "Cognitive Behavioral Therapy+" (CBT+) described by Dorsey, Berliner, Lyon, Pullmann, and Murray (2016). Each provides a systematic means for identifying a specific behavior and systematic selection of a common element for intervention. Both are supported by online clinical supports (PracticeWise and EBP Toolkit, respectively). If that is not successful, the practitioner records the behavior and intervention then systematically selects an alternative common element. Astute readers will note similarities between this and *a process of evidence-based practice*. Research on modularized approaches is promising. However, they must be implemented with clear guidelines for practice and support (typically in the form of coaching and use of data systems). These guidelines are critical to ensure that practitioners remain systematic. The danger is that practitioners will eclectically select strategies and not stick to the common elements approach. When this occurs, it is minimally effective and outcomes approximate eclectic approaches to practice.

A System of Evidence-Based Services

There are many considerations when developing or assessing the appropriateness of a system of community-based services. Communities should collaborate and carefully consider the availability of different practice models to address a variety of problems and concerns for different age groups. Are there interventions for infants and new parents? How about for toddlers and preschool-age children? How about elementary and middle school students? What about adolescents and emerging adults? Adults and the elderly? No single promising or evidence-based practice addresses behaviors and concerns across all stages of human development. Thus, identifying and implementing a suite of programs, or systems of care, is essential.

A second consideration for communities is service intensity. Ideally, prevention, early intervention, and more intensive interventions should be available. From a public health standpoint, the most intensive services should be available for those in greatest need. If a community implements sufficient and appropriate prevention and early intervention practices, then over time, there should be less need for higher intensive services.

A third consideration in developing a system of services is to provide sufficient appropriate practices to address the extent of typical behaviors and concerns in that community. Anxiety, depression, traumatic stress, behavioral problems, and substance use are the most common disorders requiring treatment. In developing a community's services, it is also important to assess the availability of specialized treatments. Although fewer people may require them, services for eating disorders, suicide, obsessive-compulsive disorders, tic disorders, and other less common maladies are necessary.

Availability is a final consideration for a community developing a system of services. Some communities may have many promising or evidence-based practices available, but an insufficient number of providers to meet the demand. It is just as important to assess the service availability for linguistically and culturally diverse children, youth, families, and adults. Finally, and practically, transportation and service location must be considered.

There are models such as Communities that Care (Hawkins, Catalano, & Kuklinski, 2014) that can guide communities to be thoughtful about building a system of services based on the unique needs of the community, as identified by key indicators such as the Healthy Youth Survey.

Summary

There are well-established practices for treatment of anxiety, traumatic stress, depression, substance use disorders, and behavioral disorders, including a "common elements" approach to address multiple disorders. However, because they are not well integrated within and between communities, there is a "science-to-practice" gap. The scientific tension between internal and external validity in clinical trials contributes to this gap. Therefore, pragmatic strategies supporting assessment of treatment fidelity are essential to develop and transport these practices into community-based settings.

References

Alexander, J., Barton, C., Gordon, D., Grotpeter, J., Hansson, K., Harrison, R., et al. (1998). *Blueprints for violence prevention, book three: Functional family therapy.* Boulder, CO: Center for the Study and Prevention of Violence.

Chorpita, B. F., Daleiden, E., & Weisz, J. R. (2005). Identifying and selecting the common elements of evidence based interventions: A distillation and matching model. *Mental Health Services Research, 7,* 5–20.

Cohen, J. A., Mannarino, A. P., & Deblinger, E. (2006). *Treating trauma and traumatic grief in children and adolescents* (2nd ed.). New York: The Guilford Press.

Dorsey, S., Berliner, L., Lyon, A. R., Pullmann, M. D., & Murray, L. K. (2016). A statewide common elements initiative for children's mental health. *The Journal of Behavioral Health Services & Research, 43*(2), 246–261.

Dorsey, S., McLaughlin, K. A., Kerns, S. E. U., Harrison, J. P., Lambert, H. K., Briggs-King, E., ... Amaya-Jackson, L. (2017). Evidence base update for psychosocial treatments for children and adolescents exposed to traumatic events. *Journal of Clinical Child and Adolescent Psychology, 46*(3), 303–330. https://doi.org/10.1080/15374416.2016.1220309.

Dorsey, S., Pullmann, M. D., Deblinger, E., Berliner, L., Kerns, S. E., Thompson, K., ... & Garland, A. F. (2013). Improving practice in community-based settings: A randomized trial of supervision—study protocol. *Implementation Science, 8*(1), 89.

Foa, E. B., Hembree, E. A., Cahill, S. P., Rauch, S. A., Riggs, D. S., Feeny, N. C., & Yadin, E. (2005). Randomized trial of prolonged exposure for posttraumatic stress disorder with and without cognitive restructuring: Outcome at academic and community clinics. *Journal of Consulting and Clinical psychology, 73*(5), 953.

Foa, E. B., Keane, T. M., Friedman, M. J., & Cohen, J. A. (Eds.). (2008). *Effective treatments for PTSD: Practice guidelines from the international society for traumatic stress studies.* Guilford Press.

Forehand, R., Dorsey, S., Jones, D. J., Long, N., & McMahon, R. J. (2010). Adherence and flexibility: They can (and do) coexist! *Clinical Psychology: Science and Practice, 17*(3), 258–264.

Funderburk, B. W., & Eyberg, S. (2011). Parent–child interaction therapy. In J. C. Norcross, G. R. VandenBos, & D. K. Freedheim (Eds.), *History of psychotherapy: Continuity and change* (pp. 415–420). Washington, DC, US: American Psychological Association.

Gregersen, E. (2010). *An explorer's guide to the universe.* Rosen Publishing Group.

Hawkins, J. D., Catalano, R. F., & Kuklinski, M. R. (2014). Communities that care. In *Encyclopedia of criminology and criminal justice* (pp. 393–408). New York, NY: Springer.

Henggeler, S. W., Schoenwald, S. K., Borduin, C. M., Rowland, M. D., & Cunningham, P. B. (2009). *Multisystemic therapy for anti-social behavior in children and adolescents* (2nd ed.). New York: Guilford Press.

Hogue, A., Henderson, C. E., Dauber, S., Barajas, P. C., Fried, A., & Liddle, H. A. (2008). Treatment adherence, competence, and outcome in individual and family therapy for adolescent behavior problems. *Journal of Consulting and Clinical Psychology, 76*(4), 544–555.

Kaminski, J. W., Valle, L. A., Filene, J. H., & Boyle, C. L. (2008). A meta-analytic review of components associated with parent training program effectiveness. *Journal of Abnormal Child Psychology, 36*(4), 567–589.

Kendall, P. C. (2006). *Coping cat workbook* (2nd ed.). Workbook Publishing.

Kendall, P. C., Crawford, E. A., Kagan, E. R., Furr, J. M., & Podell, J. L. (2003). Child-focused treatment of anxiety. In J. R. Weisz & A. E. Kazdin (Eds.), *Evidence-based psychotherapies for children and adolescents* (3rd ed., pp 81–100). Guilford Press.

Lieberman, A. F., Van Horn, P., & Ippen, C. G. (2005). Toward evidence-based treatment: Child-parent psychotherapy with preschoolers exposed to marital violence. *Journal of the American Academy of Child and Adolescent Psychiatry, 44*(12), 1241–1248.

Mazzucchelli, T. G., & Sanders, M. R. (2010). Facilitating practitioner flexibility within an empirically supported intervention: Lessons from a system of parenting support. *Clinical Psychology: Science and Practice, 17*(3), 238–252.

McMahon, R. J., & Forehand, R. L. (2005). *Helping the noncompliant child: Family-based treatment for oppositional behavior.* New York, NY: Guilford Press.

Mufson, L., & Moreau, D. (1999). Interpersonal psychotherapy for depressed adolescents (IPT-A). *Handbook of psychotherapies with children and families* (pp. 239–253). Boston, MA: Springer.

Reitman, D., & McMahon, R. J. (2013). Constance "Connie" Hanf (1917–2002): The mentor and the model. *Cognitive and Behavioral Practice, 20*(1), 106–116.

Sanders, M. R. (1999). Triple P-positive parenting program: Towards an empirically validated multilevel parenting and family support strategy for the prevention of behavior and emotional problems in children. *Clinical Child and Family Psychology Review, 2*(2), 71–90.

Saxe, G. N., Ellis, B. H., & Kaplow, J. B. (2007). *Collaborative treatment of traumatized children and teens: The trauma systems therapy approach.* New York, NY: Guilford Press.

Schoenwald, S. K. (2011). It's a bird, it's a plane, it's… fidelity measurement in the real world. *Clinical Psychology: Science and Practice, 18*(2), 142–147.

Sexton, T., & Turner, C. W. (2011). The Effectiveness of Functional Family Therapy for Youth With Behavioral Problems in a Community Practice Setting. *Couple and Family Psychology: Research and Practice, 1*(S), 3–15.

Sholomaskas, D. E., Syracuse-Siewert, G., Rounsaville, B. J., Ball, S. A., Nuro, K. F., & Carroll, K. M. (2005). We don't train in vain: A dissemination trial of three strategies of training clinicians in cognitive-behavioral therapy. *Journal of Consulting and Clinical Psychology, 73*(1), 106–115.

Webster-Stratton, C., & Reid, M. J. (2003). The incredible years parents, teachers and children training series: A multifaceted treatment approach for young children with conduct problems. In J. R. Weisz & A. E. Kazdin (Eds.), *Evidence-based psychotherapies for children and adolescents* (3rd ed., pp. 194–210).

Weisz, J. R., Moore, P. S., Southam-Gerow, M. A., Weersing, V. R., Valeri, S. M., & McCarty, C. A. (2005). *Therapist's manual PASCET: Primary and secondary control enhancement training program.* Los Angeles, CA: University of California.

Chapter 8
Implementation Science: Slowing Down to Install a Practice

Concurrent with the emergence of descriptions and debates about evidence-based practice reviewed in Chap. 3, there was an increasing emphasis on outcomes (Epstein, Kutash, & Duchnowski, 1998). The search for what works contributed to discourse about maintaining treatment model fidelity (Kutash & Rivera, 1996). In Chaps. 6 and 7, we reviewed the process of model development and the critical importance of model fidelity that establish evidence of effectiveness. The increased focus upon outcomes, fidelity, and program effectiveness became nadir for the emergence of implementation science.

> *R. Spencer Darling noted that all organizations are designed, intentionally, or unwittingly, to achieve precisely the results they get* (Fixsen, Naoom, Blase, Friedman and Wallace, 2005).
> *Most efforts to install a new practice are ultimately unsustainable. A significant contributing factor to this inability to sustain is failure to adequately consider and adjust the host environment* (Aarons et al., 2016).

Every promising practice, research-based or evidence-based practice is delivered in the context of communities and especially of organizations. What an organization does or does not do to support effective delivery of that practice with fidelity in the community context is inextricably interwoven with the decision to select and deliver any program or practice model.

Until 2005, service delivery in the context of the organization and community might be discussed in select studies or evaluations across disciplines, but there was no common language nor an implementation science through which to focus. In that year, the National Implementation Research Network (NIRN) published a seminal monograph that presented findings from a review of over 800 empirical studies spanning over three decades of efforts to improve outcomes (Fixsen et al., 2005). The literature reviewed included studies from corporate business, agribusiness, hospital and school administration, education, mental health and social services, juvenile

© Springer Nature Switzerland AG 2019
R. Bertram and S. Kerns, *Selecting and Implementing Evidence-Based Practice*,
https://doi.org/10.1007/978-3-030-11325-4_8

justice, and other human endeavors. From this meta-review, NIRN researchers identified three interrelated frameworks that support and provide guidance for effective implementation. This included identification of core components of the intervention model, identification of the drivers of effective implementation, and identification of stages of implementation. These frameworks established a common foundation and language for what is now called implementation science. As of October 2018, this seminal study has been cited in over 4000 publications.

Core Intervention Components

The framework of core components of a practice model provides a sound foundation for exploration, purposeful selection, installation, and implementation by a service organization. The intervention components include (a) client population characteristics (age, gender, race, ethnicity, behaviors of concern, and multisystem involvement or other factors that research suggests can be effectively addressed by a practice model; (b) model definition (who should be engaged in what activities, elements, and phases of service delivery); (c) theory bases supporting those elements and activities; and (d) the practice model's theory of change that describes how those elements and activities create improved outcomes for the client population. Careful consideration of these components supports the organization's alignment of implementation drivers during the installation and introduction of the new practice (Bertram, Blase, & Fixsen, 2015).

Implementation Drivers

NIRN's examination of over 800 empirical studies (Fixsen et al., 2005) identified a framework of implementation drivers that an organization can adjust to support consistent, effective delivery of a practice with fidelity. NIRN also discussed the integrated and compensatory nature of these drivers. Implementation drivers establish the organization's capacity to create and sustain practice, program, and system-level changes to achieve improved population outcomes (Bertram et al., 2015; Blase, Van Dyke, Fixsen, & Bailey, 2012).

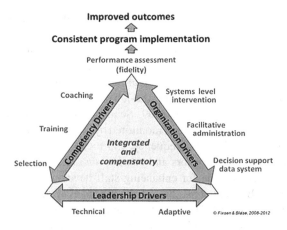

Implementation Drivers. Copyright 2008–2012 by Fixsen and Blase. Reprinted with permission

Competency drivers (staff selection, training, coaching, and performance assessment) develop staff competence and confidence to deliver the treatment model effectively and with fidelity.

Staff selection. Based upon client population characteristics and the practice model's elements and activities, criteria and processes for selecting staff should be adjusted. This should include evaluating the potential staff member's willingness and comfort in using data to improve delivery of the new practice effectively and with fidelity. It should also include their abilities to respond to and to apply coaching toward greater fidelity and effectiveness. Attitudes toward evidence-based practice and staff confidence and ability to learn something new are discussed in subsequent chapters.

Training and coaching. Successful and sustainable implementation of any practice model requires behavior change in practitioners, their supervisors or coaches, and in the administration of the host organization. Training and coaching shape and support this behavior change in carefully selected staff (Bertram et al., 2015). The most potent training focuses through the intervention component framework, so staff develop common knowledge of population characteristics and the reasons for choosing the practice model, its theory of change and research supporting its effectiveness with that population. Key elements and activities and the theory bases supporting them should be clearly understood, and there should be opportunities for practicing them in the training. Ideally training should include pre- and post-evaluations that establish a baseline to begin on-the-job coaching to support staff as they apply this new knowledge and skill. A post-training evaluation can include questions about staff confidence and ability to deliver the new practice. This can help individualize subsequent coaching. Pre- and post-training evaluations also serve as data to inform administrators about effectiveness of the training.

However, training alone is never sufficient. The initial training develops staff understanding and buy-in to the new practice. It develops initial knowledge and skills. Increasingly competent and confident use of any treatment model is most effectively developed through skillful on-the-job coaching (Henggeler, Schoenwald, Borduin, Rowland, & Cunningham, 2009; Schoenwald, Sheidow, & Letourneau, 2004). Coaching should be planned and monitored by the organization. A written plan should identify coaching formats, frequency, and focus. Fidelity and outcome data should inform coaching. Supervisors and coaches should be well selected, trained, coached, and held accountable for enhancing staff development through plan-do-study-act processes (Bertram et al., 2015; Schoenwald et al., 2004).

Performance assessment. The final competency driver is performance (fidelity) assessment. Two types of fidelity/performance data should be developed and monitored. One type of model fidelity is related to practitioner performance with clients. When examined with client outcome data, this also reflects how well the competency drivers of staff selection, training, and coaching are functioning, as well as how hospitable the environment is in promoting conditions that support high-fidelity, effective practice. This second form of performance/fidelity assessment is called organizational fidelity (Bertram et al., 2015; Schoenwald et al., 2004).

Organization drivers create practice-supportive administrative policies and procedures. Each should be aligned with the practice model and monitored. Administrators must also attend to funding and to the interface with other systems to ensure that competency drivers are effective. They should monitor population outcomes while ensuring continuous quality improvement. These drivers are not the responsibility of practitioners.

Facilitative administration. Administrators must be proactive. To achieve desired client outcomes, they must facilitate organizational change. Organization policy and procedures should be adjusted to best support and sustain program implementation. This includes adjusting and monitoring each competency driver, as well as size of caseload or other staff responsibilities. As implementation fidelity is achieved, administrators continue to facilitate and learn from model-pertinent information in practice-to-policy and policy-to-practice data feedback loops. Each implementation driver must be consistently monitored for quality and fidelity because diminished fidelity is a short path to diminished client outcomes. Working within and through implementation drivers, administrators shape organization climate and culture to accommodate and support new functions necessary to implement the program model effectively, efficiently, and with fidelity (Bertram et al., 2015; Schoenwald et al., 2004).

> *Model-pertinent data to guide administrative decisions about organizational change and fidelity of staff performance are essential for quality improvement and program sustainability.*

Decision-support data systems. Data systems should provide predetermined, valid information about fidelity and population outcomes. Data reports should be timely, consistent, and accessible to implementation teams. These teams may include practice model purveyors like the researchers in Chap. 7, as well as administrators, supervisors, and staff. The data can be very simple. For example, consistent reports on the frequency, formats, focus, and participation in coaching are easily organized for review. These data can be compared with consistent reports about practice fidelity and client outcomes to inform adjustments to competency drivers.

System-level interventions. Influenced by shifting socioeconomic, political, and cultural concerns, implementation occurs in the changing contexts of federal, state, organizational, and community factors. Practice fidelity, population outcomes, and program sustainability can be influenced by these factors. Consistent administrative monitoring of practice-to-policy and policy-to-practice information feedback is necessary to anticipate and to address challenges to effective implementation with fidelity of the program model.

For example, discussed in Chap. 3, the 2018 passage of the Family First Prevention Services Act requires child welfare organizations receiving federal funds to use effective practices and programs supported by research to prevent child abuse or neglect. As a result, adjustments will necessarily occur between state systems and private agencies serving families in which children are at risk for abuse or neglect. As new practices are adopted, organizations must adjust how their selected practice model interfaces with other organizations serving these families so that their efforts complement and do not constrain or compete with each other.

Leadership drivers. Organization leaders will face challenges as they adopt a new practice and adjust implementation drivers. They must discern whether those challenges require adaptive or technical strategies (Heifetz & Laurie, 1997). Technical leadership is appropriate in circumstances of certainty and agreement about the implementation challenge and the correct course of action. More traditional management approaches that focus on a single point of accountability using well-understood and accepted methods and processes are best used to address such implementation challenges (Daly & Chrispeels, 2008; Waters, Marzano, & McNulty, 2003). Adaptive leadership is required when there is less certainty and less agreement about the nature of problems and their solutions. Adaptive leadership strategies are needed in more complex conditions to understand a challenge and develop consensus on how to address it (Daly & Chrispeels, 2008; Waters et al., 2003). Coaching, facilitative administration, and system-level interventions are more likely to require adaptive forms of leadership to determine the nature of the challenge, to develop consensus about possible solutions and to monitor results of the problem-solving efforts (Bertram et al., 2015).

Implementation Stages

Finally, NIRN's seminal study (Fixsen et al., 2005) identified implementation stages and described the activities that occur in each stage as the organization works with staff, community stakeholders, funding sources, and treatment model purveyors to select and adopt and then to install a new practice before beginning its initial implementation with clients. Careful implementation is a process, not an event. Done well, it can take from two to four years before the new practice is fully implemented with consistent and sustainable fidelity and expected outcomes (Bertram et al., 2015).

To implement efficiently and well, NIRN recommends that organizations not rush to initiate a new practice and instead take time to carefully consider and adjust implementation drivers in a transformation zone before scaling up the practice throughout an organization or system. Although the figure below may visually imply a linear progression through stages of implementation, changes in funding, leadership, socioeconomic conditions, staff turnover, or other events may require the organization to readdress activities of earlier stages of implementation. For a thorough discussion of NIRN stages of implementation, see Bertram et al. (2015), and Fixsen et al. (2005). A brief summary of these stages are as follows.

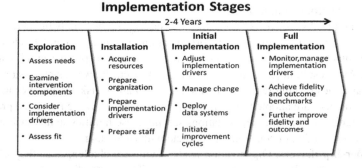

Implementation Stages. Bertram, Blase, and Fixsen (2015)

Exploration. Also called "exploration and adoption," in this stage the organization carefully examines target population characteristics, organization and community resources, and the program model's intervention components. This process can include an implementation team of staff and community stakeholders. Funding requirements, staffing patterns, sources of referrals as well as necessary organizational changes should be considered. This exploration process should identify the appropriateness and potential benefits of the potential new program and an explicit plan with tasks and timelines to facilitate effective and efficient installation and implementation. Proactive, small adjustments in this stage reap great benefits. Less thorough exploration amplifies subsequent challenges as the program is installed and implemented.

Installation. In this stage, the previously described competency and organizational drivers must be aligned with the new practice to support effective service delivery with fidelity. Working with purveyors, intermediary organizations (see subsequent chapters, especially Chaps. 11 and 12), and implementation-informed faculty, the implementation team should systematically examine and align each implementation driver. For example, model-pertinent criteria for staff selection, training, coaching, as well as for fidelity and outcome assessment should be clarified. Previously discussed data-informed feedback loops should be designed to refine policies and procedures. Explicit understandings between service organizations or funding sources may be necessary. Similar to the exploration stage, proactive adjustments in this stage reap great benefits.

Initial implementation. In this stage, the new practice is delivered to clients. It is a time of excitement, concern, and uncertainty. Unanticipated challenges may emerge as changes in roles, responsibilities, and practices begin. Natural discomfort with change can combine with the complexity of implementing something different to test confidence in delivery of the new practice. In the final chapters of this book, we discuss the use of transformation zones to create a limited context for organizational learning and refinement prior to scaling the new practice across the entire organization or system. With the support of well-composed and informed implementation teams, adaptive leadership normalizes challenges, and employs efficient data-informed problem solving.

Full implementation. As implementation challenges are reconciled and the new practice is scaled up from the learning environment of a transformation zone, continuous use of data feedback loops will support most practitioners to deliver the new practice with fidelity and achieve expected client outcomes. Full implementation occurs when implementation drivers are easily accessible and are regularly reviewed for continuous quality improvement.

Summary of NIRN Frameworks

NIRN's 2005 study tapped a wellspring of thought about how to improve the development and testing of an innovative practice to prove its efficacy and effectiveness, as well as its subsequent dissemination to other settings. This contributed to the emergence of a biennial Global Implementation Conference and similar conferences in Australia, Scandinavia, and Canada concurrent with the emergence of a journal called *Implementation Science*. In these forums, researchers, policymakers, purveyors, and practitioners present their experiences, questions, and studies that focus upon the process of developing, disseminating, and implementing evidence-based practice.

Selecting a practice proven to be effective with a client population is simply the first of many steps an organization must take to deliver that practice in a sustainable, effective manner with fidelity. Slowing down to carefully align implementation drivers and to consider a range of strategies and approaches is time well spent toward successful installation and initial implementation of that practice.

In the remaining portions of this chapter, we review approaches that focus through implementation science to facilitate adjustments to inner and outer setting factors to support sustainable implementation of proven practices. We briefly review Damschroder et al., (2009) framework for implementation as well as some practical approaches informed by Powell et al., (2015) and colleagues' taxonomy of implementation support strategies. We also explore the "adaptable periphery" of implementation. These aspects are flexible and can be adapted based on organizational context, community culture, and practitioner factors.

Implementation and Context

Now, that you are familiar with implementation science and frameworks, let us extrapolate from the Chap. 6 example of how an innovative practice is tested and proven effective. Imagine that the *effectiveness trial* was presented at a national conference. In the audience were representatives from a federal grant site in another state who approached the model developer. This site was unsuccessful in efforts to improve outcomes for the age group of children that the researcher's new evidence-based practice so successfully addressed. The site leaders explained that in the final year of their grant, remaining funds had to be spent and expressed strong interest in learning to provide the researcher's evidence-based practice.

Although there were only nine months remaining in the grant, the researcher and the behavioral healthcare organization quickly organized a three-day training event for fifteen practitioners and two supervisors responsible for services to improve outcomes for families with children aged five to twelve years old. The training event presented the studies and their outcomes, as well as key elements and activities of the researcher's evidence-based practice. Participants in the training seemed excited to try the new practice. The researcher emphasized that to improve child and family outcomes, the supervisors should review videotapes of practitioner–family sessions. However, the quickly planned training provided no time for supervisors to be coached by the researcher on how to review videotapes and use it with practitioners to improve their competence and confidence.

Two months after the training, administrator and supervisors called the researcher. Only eight of the practitioners had used the intervention with any families, and of those eight, several reported challenges getting families to complete treatment sessions. The researcher asked what contributed to this, but neither the administrator nor the supervisors had systematically gathered data about this challenge. Instead, they shared anecdotal stories from practitioners that seemed to be unique to each family.

Probing further, the researcher asked if, in their review of videotaped sessions, the supervisors identified possible contributing factors to families not completing the treatment sessions. There was a poignant moment of silence. Finally, a supervisor shared that there were only a few videotapes to review. He believed practitioners were not used to being videotaped and suspected that some were not asking for family permission. He stated that other practitioners complained that their caseload was too high to allow time to secure family permission and then to set up and review the videotape.

Lacking systematic data and with the grant soon to expire, the researcher encouraged the supervisors to pick one of the videotapes in which the practitioner delivered the practice model with more confidence and to bring all the trained practitioners to watch it while the supervisor applauded what the clinician did well and made suggestions how it could be better. She asked the administrator to speak with all staff about the importance of securing more families to be videotaped, so supervisors could help the practitioners to feel more confident and comfortable.

Four months later, and six months after the training, only twelve families completed all sessions of the new evidence-based practice, and their outcomes were not as good as those the researcher achieved in the efficacy, effectiveness, and dissemination studies. The administrator and supervisors again joined the researcher in a conference call. They pondered what contributed to this, but the administrator and supervisors again lacked systematically gathered data, only anecdotal stories from the practitioners that seemed to be unique to each family. A few more practitioners had secured family permission to videotape sessions, but most practitioners preferred to do what they always had done and found their supervisor when he or she was free for ad hoc discussions about delivery of the new evidence-based practice. Supervisors freely discussed their many additional responsibilities that made it more difficult to schedule group coaching that used session videotapes.

> Dorsey et al. (2017) *examined what happens during the course of usual supervision, even when an agency is trying to implement an evidence-based practice. In this study, 207 clinicians and 56 supervisors were implementing Trauma-Focused Cognitive Behavior Therapy (TF-CBT). This study found that clinicians usually received weekly supervision. However, about 20% of this time was spent on administrative and other concerns. In fact, only about 20 min of a supervision hour was dedicated to the two most important clinical functions, namely case conceptualization and the activities and elements of TF-CBT.*

How did this happen? And how could this be prevented in the future? From the researcher/treatment developer perspective, the concerns may focus on the community's and behavioral healthcare center's inability to replicate conditions present during the effectiveness and dissemination trials. There had been no engagement and preparation of the community to excite family interest. Both practitioner caseload and supervisor responsibilities to ensure completion of billing to insurance providers were problematic. From the community or family perspective, this innovative evidence-based practice seemed to be a somewhat intrusive intervention that required them to find time to get away from work and bring their child from school for the sessions. Many experienced it as ineffective and sensed discomfort or lack of confidence in the practitioner, so they simply stopped participating. Indeed, after only three days of training, many of the practitioners were not comfortable or confident. Supervisors themselves were not as comfortable or confident as the researcher in reviewing videotapes with practitioners. They complained about how much time they had to spend reviewing videotapes to prepare to coach practitioners using videotape review. Everyone seemed frustrated and disappointed.

A Formula for Success

Why would the innovative evidence-based practice developed by the researcher in Chap. 6 achieve such good results in the lab efficacy trial and in the initial effectiveness trial but not readily transport to another community setting? In NIRN's graphic equation, *Formula for Success*, Metz & Barley (2012) visually highlight the necessary relationships between effective implementation that supports delivery of an effective practice in an enabling context. If any portion of this formula is zero (missing), expected outcomes cannot be achieved.

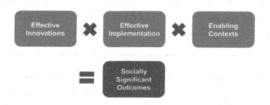

Effective Innovations. In the process of establishing the effectiveness of an innovative, promising practice, it is essential to examine characteristics of the practice and the extent to which it is appropriate for the population of concern in the community. In Chap. 6, the practice model was tested for families with children aged five to twelve years old. It was also tested in a specific geographic area with its own unique community demographics and cultural composition. However, all too often an agency may extend delivery of the practice to older children, only to discover that it may not be effective for adolescents.

There could be ways that the structure of an effective practice constrains its transportability across cultures. Take the example of Parent–Child Interaction Therapy (PCIT), developed by Sheila Eyberg (Funderbuck & Eyberg, 2011). This intervention is traditionally delivered to families with children between the ages of two and seven who have disruptive behavior problems. Practitioners are trained clinicians who administer PCIT in a clinic-based setting. They watch from behind a one-way mirror as the parents apply elements and activities of PCIT with their children. The clinician then uses a bug-in-the-ear strategy to coach parents as they engage their children. PCIT is highly effective in treating behavior problems for this age group (Eyberg et al., 2001). However, there was recognition that PCIT needed adaptations to be optimally effective for Native American and Alaskan Native populations. Dee

Bigfoot and colleagues created a cultural adaptation called Honoring Children, Making Relatives (BigFoot & Funderburk, 2011). In this adaptation, several clinical and implementation changes made PCIT more culturally appropriate. Their article provides excellent details and case examples of the clinical adaptation, which strived to maintain the essence of PCIT while incorporating concepts, context, and conceptualizations of Native culture. Further, from an implementation standpoint, this adaptation uses dissemination strategies that are more consistent with the realities of more rural service delivery. This included being more flexible about practitioner credentials, training, and coaching supports, as well as incorporating telehealth strategies to reach remote families. While this demonstrates a responsive adaptation of an effective program, there are no published studies of this specific adaptation. And, this is not an uncommon conundrum. Many adaptations are not evaluated, and as a result, we do not know how effective they are. The need to explore adaptations highlights the important point that an intervention that is effective in one context or with a certain group may or may not be effective in a different context.

Effective Implementation. There are several different ways that implementation can compromise client outcomes. In this chapter's extrapolated example, there was little time to plan installation of the new evidence-based practice in the behavioral healthcare organization. The organization and the researcher/treatment purveyor focused on organizing the three-day training event. This is unfortunately all too common. Although the use of session videotapes as a format and focus for supervision was introduced, there was insufficient time or attention in those three days for the supervisors and the practitioners to practice using videotape in this manner. More importantly, there was no exploration and discussion with them and with the administrator about caseload and other responsibilities that might constrain using videotapes to improve practitioner competence and confidence, nor did they explore staff concerns about being videotaped.

With the advent of implementation science and frameworks, researchers can now anticipate all of these potential challenges and more. Implementation research has articulated a number of important steps and considerations that should be taken before starting to deliver new practices. This may take months or even a year. Organizations must "slow down to speed up." The organization must slow down to install a new practice by adjusting implementation drivers to create staff understanding, support, and confidence before initial delivery of the practice with clients.

Careful installation of new practice sustains and supports its effective implementation. The researcher/purveyor and the administrator and supervisors in this chapter's extrapolated example did not establish a referral pathway (*systems-level interventions*), nor carefully consider caseload and other responsibilities (*facilitative administration*), nor did they establish data systems to consistently monitor frequency, formats, and focus of supervision (data systems are further discussed in Chap. 11).

After introducing the new practice in the three-day training event, when practitioners did not receive timely appropriate referrals, there could have been a loss of enthusiasm for the new evidence-based practice. Further, protracted lengths of time between training and practice can lead to degradation in learning or in practitioner confidence. When families were referred, this degradation of knowledge or confidence could have created a disincentive for the practitioner to complete a permission forms to videotape the family sessions.

Another potential implementation challenge was maintaining practice fidelity when few families completed all of the treatment sessions, and fewer still were videotaped and reviewed with the supervisor. Anecdotal stories from practitioners to their supervisor identified the size of their caseload and other responsibilities as limiting time to secure family permission, to set up the videotape, to provide it to the supervisor, and then make time to review it later with the supervisor. One supervisor thought that perhaps because the clinicians were uncomfortable, the families were uncomfortable and so did not complete all sessions, thus completing a negative feedback loop of fewer families, fewer videotaped sessions, and limited time for supervisors and practitioners to prepare for and to review videotapes. Compromised video review compromised fidelity and staff competence and confidence. Perhaps, families sensed this and did not participate in all sessions, and so on. Without monitoring treatment fidelity, we have no way of knowing if poor outcomes have something to do with the intervention itself or with the implementation of the intervention by the practitioners or by the organization.

Enabling Contexts. How supportive is the context for the process of learning to deliver a new practice? Does leadership fully understand and support this? How do the policies and procedures of the organization align with the new practice? Does the culture of the organization and its interface with the community support a "problem-solving" state of mind? Some organizations have naturally adaptive and enabling contexts. For others, the climate, culture, and sometimes structures must be adapted to enable effective implementation. In this chapter's extrapolated example, the organization was not achieving desired client outcomes before it heard the researcher's conference presentation. They assumed the problem was due to the practices they were delivering through the grant. However, even the new evidence-based practice was not well-implemented. Its effectiveness was compromised by failure to carefully consider its installation, including outreach to inform the community about it.

The researcher/purveyor in our extrapolated example did not have knowledge or substantive experience with implementation science. This is not uncommon among treatment developers. When true, a purveyor must partner with someone who does understand implementation science to help the service organization develop an implementation plan. Intermediary organizations often play this role and can be effective partners in this space (Franks & Bory, 2015). There will be further discussion of these organizations in Chap. 12.

Other Frameworks for Implementation

Since publication of NIRN's seminal study (Fixsen et al., 2005), research about implementation has contributed to articulation of means to guide service agencies and intermediary organizations in successful implementation. A review by Tabak,

Khoong, Chambers, and Brownson (2012) identified 61 different models for improving implementation. A recent scoping review of knowledge translation theories by Strifler et al. (2018) identified 159, but 60% of the frameworks, models, or theories for implementation research were used only once. In this burgeoning literature about implementation, there currently appear to be five main categories of discussion: process models, determinant frameworks, classic theories, implementation theories, and evaluation frameworks (Nilsen, 2015). Each offers different descriptions, but none are unanimously endorsed.

A frequently used process model, the "Consolidated Framework for Implementation Research" (CFIR), was articulated by Damschroder and colleagues in 2009. A systematic review of the use of CFIR in implementation research conducted between August 2009 and January 2015 found 429 unique peer-reviewed articles that used it (Kirk et al., 2015). By mid-2018, according to Google Scholar, the CFIR has been cited in over 2850 articles.

The CFIR somewhat overlaps but then extends the NIRN formula for success. It identifies five domains that impact implementation: intervention characteristics, outer setting, inner setting, characteristics of the individuals involved, and the process of implementation (Damschroder et al., 2009). Astute readers will note that intervention characteristics appear similar to NIRN's framework of intervention components. An important contribution that CFIR makes is articulating the difference between an intervention's core components (i.e., "the active ingredients", the elements and activities that should not change) and its "adaptable periphery." The adaptable periphery are those elements of the intervention that can be altered without compromising the core components. These changes may be necessary to embed the intervention within a unique context (e.g., translating practice model elements and activities to Spanish as occurred in the Chap. 6 dissemination study).

The outer setting are systemic factors that impact implementation. This can include broader sociopolitical impacts as well as more proximal systemic impacts such as healthcare funding structures. This is similar to systems-level interventions in the NIRN framework of implementation drivers.

The inner setting is more specific to the characteristics of the agency itself, including how it is structured and governed, the policies, procedures, and practices that help shape the overall agency culture and climate. This is similar to facilitative administration and its adjustment of data systems and competency drivers in the NIRN framework of implementation drivers.

Characteristics of individuals include participants' attitudes, power, personal agency, skills, and beliefs. There has been significant research on this part of CFIR's process of implementation model. For example, many studies show that baseline positive attitudes toward evidence-based practices are predictive of successful implementation (e.g., Aarons & Sawitzky, 2006; Kerns et al., 2017).

Finally, while taking into consideration the inner and outer contexts in which implementation is occurring, CFIR describes the process of implementation as a key dynamic that helps create a fit between the selected practice model and the setting. This process can happen in sequential stages or as an iterative process. This is similar to the NIRN discussion of implementation stages.

Implementation Strategies

While CFIR facilitates consideration of the complex interrelationships between factors influencing implementation, it is helpful to have strategies to address specific implementation goals. Powell et al. (2012) compiled 68 different implementation strategies and then updated and refined the list to contain 73 different strategies in Powell et al., (2015). Each strategy occurs in different implementation stages and addresses different implementation drivers.

- Planning: for example, conduct a community needs assessment; develop a systematic implementation blueprint; model and simulate change (*exploration and adoption; installation stages*).

- Educating: for example, conduct educational outreach with agency partners and referral sources; conduct initial and ongoing training and coaching (*system-level interventions; training; coaching*) (*stages of exploration and installation*).

- Financing: for example, access new funding; finance and contract with practice model experts; align and simplify billing procedures (*facilitative administration; system-level interventions*) (*stages of exploration and installation*).

- Restructuring: for example, align case data systems; create new clinical teams (*facilitative administration; decision-making data systems; coaching*) (*installation and initial implementation stages*).

- Ensuring quality: for example, develop and apply fidelity assessment tools; align organizational fidelity monitoring procedures (*facilitative administration; decision-making data systems; coaching*) (*installation; initial implementation; full implementation stages*).

- Attending to the policy context: for example, change liability laws; inform and align advisory boards or community workgroups (*facilitative administration; system-level interventions*) (*all stages*).

For example, focusing through the NIRN drivers, an agency may recognize that policies and procedures must be aligned with the new practice model (*facilitative administration*). Administrators, managers, and their implementation team would then review these strategies and determine which of the other implementation drivers require similar alignment to sustain effective implementation of the new practice with fidelity. Within the CFIR, these strategies may be helpful when inner or outer context challenges impact implementation. Outer context policies frequently present challenges to effective implementation. A common occurrence encountered during implementation planning is when Medicaid billing procedures and reimbursement rates are not favorable for the preferred new practice model. The practice model may require a range of activities or resources that are not directly billable to Medicaid. This can create a substantial financial burden, and the organization may determine that the preferred practice model is not feasible to implement. However, if there are strong policy partners, local Medicaid providers may advocate for higher reimbursement rates or case rates that support that diverse range of activities and resources. This is an example of the NIRN implementation driver *system-level interventions.*

Summary

The process of implementation is rarely linear. It requires careful attention to stages of implementation and the drivers that impact implementation. This takes time and effort before delivery of the new practice with clients. However, when implemented poorly, even stellar interventions are unlikely to achieve outcomes promised by the research. A thorough selection and implementation process that is responsive to the community and organizational context is invaluable. Using an established implementation framework will provide a blueprint for this process (Tabak et al., 2012), while matching implementation strategies to known needs will ensure a comprehensive approach (Powell et al., 2015).

References

Aarons, G. A., Green, A. E., Trott, E., Willging, C. E., Torres, E. M., Ehrhart, M. G., & Roesch, S. C. (2016). The roles of system and organizational leadership in system-wide evidence-based intervention sustainment: A mixed-method study. *Administration and Policy in Mental Health and Mental Health Services Research, 43*(6), 991–1008.

Aarons, G. A., & Sawitzky, A. C. (2006). Organizational culture and climate and mental health provider attitudes toward evidence-based practice. *Psychological Services, 3*(1), 61.

Bertram, R. M., Blase, K. A., & Fixsen, D. L. (2015). Improving programs and outcomes: Implementation frameworks and organization change. *Research on Social Work Practice, 25*(4), 477–487.

BigFoot, D. S., & Funderburk, B. W. (2011). Honoring children, making relatives: The cultural translation of parent–child interaction therapy for American Indian and Alaska Native families. *Journal of Psychoactive Drugs, 43*(4), 309–318.

Blase, K. A., Van Dyke, M., Fixsen, D. L., & Bailey, F. W. (2012). Implementation science: Key concepts, themes, and evidence for practitioners in educational psychology. In B. Kelly & D. Perkins (Eds.), *Handbook of implementation science for psychology in education* (pp. 13–34). London: Cambridge University Press.

Daly, A. J., & Chrispeels, J. (2008). A question of trust: Predictive conditions for adaptive and technical leadership in educational contexts. *Leadership and Policy in Schools, 7*(1), 30–63.

Damschroder, L. J., Aron, D. C., Keith, R. E., Kirsh, S. R., Alexander, J. A., & Lowery, J. C. (2009). Fostering implementation of health services research findings into practice: A consolidated framework for advancing implementation science. *Implementation science, 4*(1), 50.

Dorsey, S., Pullmann, M. D., Kerns, S. E., Jungbluth, N., Meza, R., Thompson, K., & Berliner, L. (2017). The juggling act of supervision in community mental health: Implications for supporting evidence-based treatment. *Administration and Policy in Mental Health and Mental Health Services Research, 44*(6), 838–852.

Epstein, M. H., Kutash, K., & Duchnowski, A. (Eds.). (1998). *Outcomes for children and youth with emotional and behavioral disorders and their families: Programs and evaluation best practices*. Austin, TX: PRO-ED.

Eyberg, S. M., Funderburk, B. W., Hembree-Kigin, T. L., McNeil, C. B., Querido, J. G., & Hood, K. K. (2001). Parent–child interaction therapy with behavior problem children: One and two year maintenance of treatment effects in the family. *Child & Family Behavior Therapy, 23*(4), 1–20.

Fixsen, D. L., Naoom, S. F., Blase, K. A., Friedman, R. M., & Wallace, F. (2005). *Implementation research: A synthesis of the literature*. Tampa, FL: University of South Florida, Louis de la Parte Florida Mental Health Institute, The National Implementation Research Network (FMHI Publication #231).

Franks, R. P., & Bory, C. T. (2015). Who supports the successful implementation and sustainability of evidence-based practices? Defining and understanding the roles of intermediary and purveyor organizations. *New Directions for Child and Adolescent Development, 149*, 41–56.

Funderburk, B. W., & Eyberg, S. (2011). Parent–child interaction therapy. In J. C. Norcross, G. R. VandenBos, & D. K. Freedheim (Eds.), *History of psychotherapy: Continuity and change* (pp. 415–420). Washington, DC, US: American Psychological Association.

Heifetz, R. A., & Laurie, D. L. (1997). The work of leadership. *Harvard Business Review, 75*, 124–134.

Henggeler, S. W., Schoenwald, S. K., Borduin, C. M., Rowland, M. D., & Cunningham, P. B. (2009). *Multisystemic therapy for anti-social behavior in children and adolescents* (2nd ed.). New York: Guilford Press.

Kerns, S. E. U., McCormick, E., Negrete, A., Carey, C., Haaland, W., & Waller, S. (2017). Predicting post-training implementation of a parenting intervention. *Journal of Children's Services, 12*(4), 302–315.

Kirk, M. A., Kelley, C., Yankey, N., Birken, S. A., Abadie, B., & Damschroder, L. (2015). A systematic review of the use of the consolidated framework for implementation research. *Implementation Science, 11*(1), 72.

Kutash, K., & Rivera, V. R. (1996). *What works in children's mental health services?: Uncovering answers to critical questions* (Vol. 3). Paul H Brookes Publishing Company.

Metz, A., & Bartley, L. (2012). Active implementation frameworks for program success: How to use implementation science to improve outcomes for children. *Zero to Three Journal, 34*(4), 11–18.

Nilsen, P. (2015). Making sense of implementation theories, models and frameworks. *Implementation Science, 10*(1), 53.

Powell, B. J., McMillen, J. C., Proctor, E. K., Carpenter, C. R., Griffey, R. T., Bunger, A. C., … & York, J. L. (2012). A compilation of strategies for implementing clinical innovations in health and mental health. *Medical Care Research and Review, 69*(2), 123–157.

Powell, B. J., Waltz, T. J., Chinman, M. J., Damschroder, L. J., Smith, J. L., Matthieu, M. M., … & Kirchner, J. E. (2015). A refined compilation of implementation strategies: Results from the Expert Recommendations for Implementing Change (ERIC) project. *Implementation Science, 10*(1), 21.

Schoenwald, S. K., Sheidow, A. J., & Letourneau, E. J. (2004). Toward effective quality assurance in evidence-based practice: Links between expert consultation, therapist fidelity, and child outcomes. *Journal of Clinical Child and Adolescent Psychology, 33*(1), 94–104.

Strifler, L., Cardoso, R., McGowan, J., Cogo, E., Nincic, V., Khan, P. A., … & Treister, V. (2018). Scoping review identifies significant number of knowledge translation theories, models, and frameworks with limited use. *Journal of Clinical Epidemiology, 100*, 92–102.

Tabak, R. G., Khoong, E. C., Chambers, D. A., & Brownson, R. C. (2012). Bridging research and practice: Models for dissemination and implementation research. *American Journal of Preventive Medicine, 43*(3), 337–350.

Waters, T., Marzano, R. J., & McNulty, B. (2003). Balanced leadership: What 30 years of research tells us about the effect of leadership on student achievement. A working paper. Retrieved from https://eric.ed.gov/?id=ED481972.

Chapter 9
Starting Small: Transformation Zones and Initial Implementation

Imagine an organization is completing exploration and adoption and installation stage activities and schedules a training event. This is a very exciting time. Hopes are high. If done well, this is the culmination of prerequisite activities needed before engaging clients in the evidence-based service. However, to enhance efficiency and success, it is important to begin initial implementation in a small portion of the organization, a transformation zone, where many of the common concerns discussed in this chapter can be experienced, learned from, and addressed before scaling up the new practice to include all staff.

Training

Introducing a new practice is no small undertaking. Fortunately, there is substantial research to guide the development of a successful training environment. This research can be loosely divided into three phases: pre-training preparation, initial training, and post-training supports.

Prior to training, it is critical that those who will participate understand and are invested in the idea of doing something different and have a positive attitude toward the new practice. There may be no greater challenge to effective training than to hear from participants that they had no idea why they were there, or that they were "voluntold" to be there. As you can imagine, this presents substantial implementation challenges and reduces the likelihood that these participants will be fully engaged in the learning environment. Enhanced training outcomes occur when practitioners clearly understand how a new practice better addresses client needs and outcomes. In addition to understanding this rationale, more favorable attitudes toward evidence-based practices are related to the development of competencies and confidence (self-efficacy) in the new practice. For example, six months after a Triple P-Positive Parenting Program training, practitioner attitudes toward evidence-based practice and their sense of efficacy significantly distinguished between those who delivered that evidence-based practice and those who did not (Kerns et al., 2017).

© Springer Nature Switzerland AG 2019
R. Bertram and S. Kerns, *Selecting and Implementing Evidence-Based Practice*,
https://doi.org/10.1007/978-3-030-11325-4_9

Pre-training staff preparation. How do you identify appropriate practitioners, supervisors, and managers and motivate them adequately for training? There are strategies for improving excitement and enthusiasm about a new evidence-based practice. Organizational interventions, such as Partnering For Success (Julian, 2006), Getting to Outcomes (Wandersman, Imm, Chinman, & Kaftarian, 2000), and Communities that Care (Hawkins, Catalano, & Kuklinski, 2014), can be applied within communities or organizations to identify needs in a manner that is transparent to staff and community stakeholders while engaging their perspectives and opinions. These approaches can use a multimethod process that begins with surveys, usually in combination with some examination of services frequently provided. Community surveys identify and prioritize behaviors of concern. Staff surveys explore behaviors of concern that additional training or other practices might better address. Survey results are presented to the community and to staff and identified gaps are summarized.

Then, various evidence-based practices to strategically address the identified gaps can be explored. This process empowers communities and staff and engenders hope about a new practice. Ensuring that staff know and understand administrative efforts made during the exploration and adoption or installation stages to support the use of the intervention is important to develop investment in the new practice. For example, administrators and managers can streamline case documentation. They can adopt and clarify the focus, formats, and schedules for model-pertinent supervision or consultation. They can work within the organization or with other service systems to identify and clarify means to secure appropriate client referrals.

Organization leadership should anticipate and develop plans to address any staff who express resistance or skepticism about the new practice model. This can include extra time spent clarifying the process and rationale for selection of the practice. They should be prepared to clarify and discuss staff responsibilities, how new coaching supports will help staff develop competence and confidence, and how efforts with clients will be more satisfying. Occasionally, the introduction of a new practice results in some resignations. However, if previous practices were not as effective as desired, and if staff have been fully informed about the process of selection and the alignment of supports for the new practice, then resignations may be an unfortunate but necessary process to ensure a healthy climate and culture within the organization.

Qualities of successful training. Ensuring an adequate and successful initial transfer of knowledge is critical. The initial training should be viewed as the first steps of knowledge transfer. However, training alone is not sufficient to develop staff competence and confidence in a new practice (Beidas, Barmish, & Kendall, 2009). Training without adjusting other implementation drivers is known as the "train and hope" means for knowledge transfer. Staff are trained in the hope they will do something different. Rarely is this sufficient. This point will be further developed later in this chapter. Here, we focus on how to make the initial training event as meaningful as possible.

During training, it is helpful to follow a four-step process when teaching any critical skills to enhance knowledge transfer. Step 1 is to describe the skill. It is important to provide the rationale for the skill and its function in the new practice model's theory of change. When staff develop a deep understanding of the rationale for enacting the elements and activities of the new practice model, it is more likely that clients will be engaged with fidelity (Carroll et al., 2007). This is particularly important because staff always walk a line between model fidelity and the flexibility needed to individualize model elements and activities to the clients' context. Being grounded in the theory of change helps practitioners know if potential adaptations may adversely impact the effectiveness of the practice model.

For example, a primary behavioral pattern that maintains depression is withdrawal from social activities. As individuals with depression increasingly withdraw from things that previously brought joy and positive experiences, this further increases the depressed mood. Interrupting this sequence is the essential premise for Behavioral Activation Therapy. Recall Tameisha's experiences in chapter two—depressive symptoms were reflected in the statement that her "zest for life had diminished." Her withdrawal symptoms included "missing class to go to the nurse's office," and "stopping her sports activities."

Behavioral Activation Therapy specifically identifies strategies for a client to have positive experiences and works to identify any cognition in the way of a client following through with engaging in these experiences. Because of Tameisha's academic and classroom behavioral concerns, Multisystemic Therapy was prioritized as the treatment of choice. Although not specifically a behavioral activation protocol, some features of her intervention were aligned with the principles of behavior activation, including re-engaging her in sports and social activities. This was done with the active engagement and support of her parents with the school.

Step two in effective training is to demonstrate the actual skill, and in some practice models, how to teach it to clients. It is important that trainees see an example of how to enact the activity or element of the new practice model. This starts by seeing how it is done. This typically occurs through live demonstration (e.g., modeling) or video. Ideally, this demonstrates the precise technique in a practical example. Some programs encourage practicing the skill to become familiar with how to enact it and then generate experience doing it with clients before assisting others' learning. For example, personal practice in mindfulness is a recommendation to develop the competence needed to teach mindfulness-based therapy techniques (Crane et al., 2012). Regardless, having opportunities during training to learn how to do the skill is important for adult learning. It is best to avoid more difficult client situations at this point in training. Save those scenarios for step four (training for generalization).

Step three for effective training provides participants the opportunity to practice the skill themselves within the safety of the training environment. Then, it is important that participants have the opportunity to practice teaching that skill with either a hypothetical or actual client and receive targeted feedback (e.g., role-play). A useful strategy breaks trainees into groups of three. One person is the practitioner, one the "client," and one the observer. They rotate roles during role-play so that each gets an opportunity to teach the skill and have the skill taught to them. Having an observer helps keep the role-play on task and within time allocations while also providing opportunity for objective feedback. The trainer should spend time with each group and get a sense of how well each trainee is picking up the skills. This type of behavioral feedback has been shown to be helpful in promoting treatment fidelity and can even be incorporated into supervision (e.g., Dorsey et al., 2013).

Finally, step 4 addresses potential challenges to generalization. In this step, a trainer invites participants to identify potential challenges to apply this activity and skill with clients, as well as to anticipate challenges clients might experience when they apply this activity or skill at home. This step helps practitioners anticipate challenges to treatment fidelity. During this step, the trainer demonstrates effective strategies to address common implementation conundrums. The following topics are very useful to problem-solve with trainees:

- Engagement difficulties, including clients not showing up for sessions, perpetually being late for sessions, and not completing homework;

- Investment difficulties, such as when there is evidence of limited investment in the new practice. This is often called resistance. However, resistance is usually a window into what the organization and practitioner should consider doing differently;

- Cultural considerations, including when a client's cultural beliefs may create some difficulty using the new practice;

- Process challenges, including when treatment seems to be taking longer than expected, needing to address crises that distract from treatment progress, parent, or client cognitive difficulties, etc.

Trainings are more productive when staff are prompted to carefully consider how to prevent these challenges from happening. As they consider strategies for managing such challenges as they arise, trainees should list any concerns about what could go wrong. Then, dividing trainees into small groups, each group considers how to address specific concerns to prevent them from happening, as well as strategies for how to manage the situation if it does happen. When each group shares their strategies, trainees possess multiple ideas for managing the most common clinical challenges. This increases trainee self-efficacy, and they are more likely to deliver and support the practice (e.g., Kerns et al., 2017). The following are practical examples of these topics to proactively address in this manner:

- The client is perpetually 5–15 min late for the session but always seems to have a reasonable explanation (e.g., bus was late; child refused to put seat belt on; babysitter didn't show up).

- The client asks personal questions of the therapist at every session (e.g., do you have kids? What year did you graduate high school? What is your favorite restaurant?).

- The client always seems to have a reason why the new skill or strategy will not work for them (hard to find a technique that they are motivated and willing to try).

- The client has a belief system that is counter to the therapeutic approach (e.g., they are participating in a parenting practice model, but they have a belief of "spare the rod, spoil the child").

- The client is convinced that a problem can be completely solved by dietary changes and is disinterested in hearing about cognitive or behavioral strategies.

- The client reports that their spouse or parents are not supportive of the practice.

- The client is mandated to participate and only engages to get "credit" for attending while not participating in any therapeutic activities.

- The practitioner learns the client is engaging in behaviors toward their children that require reporting neglect or abuse.

Consultation, Coaching, and Fidelity

Since training alone is never sufficient to develop new knowledge and apply new skills, there must be consistent post-training support. Lyon, Stirman, Kerns, and Bruns (2011) reviewed several different strategies to enhance post-training implementation. Two of the more evidence-based approaches include *academic detailing* (Tan, 2002) and *coaching* (Schoenwald, Sheidow, & Letourneau, 2004). Academic detailing occurs when a treatment expert meets with the trained practitioners and supervisors in their work setting. During this visit, the treatment expert observes treatment delivery and supervision then provides appropriate guidance. Although academic detailing is most often used in medical settings, it is an emerging practice to support effective implementation of evidence-based practices with fidelity. A much more common approach is coaching. Treatment experts, supervisors, or peers who are well-versed and experienced in the new practice can provide coaching. Typically, coaching occurs after live or audio/videotaped observation.

Consultation calls in which practitioners or supervisors describe implementation to a treatment expert is a common strategy widely used to support delivery of evidence-based practices with fidelity. Many practice models require six months to one year of consultation calls for certification (e.g., TF-CBT, SafeCare) while others require ongoing consultation (e.g., Multisystemic Therapy). Consultation and coaching provide a valuable means to support practitioners, supervisors, and managers to learn to sustain high-fidelity implementation of the practice model.

An interesting study by Smith-Boydston, Holtzman, and Roberts (2014) investigated what happens when practitioners delivering Multisystemic Therapy (MST) go from receiving intensive fidelity supports to no longer receiving those supports. This study is a tale of a community-based health center. Initially, the center ensured that the MST practitioners received full support for their MST implementation for three years. This included participation in weekly consultation calls, quarterly training boosters, collection of the MST Therapist Adherence Measure (TAM) to track fidelity, and other supports.

However, this agency lost funding and decided that they could not continue this level of support for MST. They continued to deliver MST, but did not participate in any of the quality assurance and improvement activities. As a result, the agency was no longer a licensed MST provider.

Although the agency endeavored to provide similar supports, some changes started to occur. The average age of the youth served decreased from 15.1 to 13.5. Also, the severity of youths' pre-treatment behavior decreased. This is important because prior research shows that MST is most effective for those youth with the most substantial problems. The agency observed that there was a substantial decrease in practitioner family contacts (from 124.6 to 66.3). Perhaps most importantly, the researchers found that for those youth who received full MST supports, there was a dramatic decrease in pre-treatment to post-treatment court-related charges (average of 1.7 charges to .55 charges). However, for youth who received MST without those fidelity supports, there were essentially no changes in pre-treatment and post-treatment court-related charges (average of .81 charges to .86 charges).

Studies such as this sound a profound cautionary note. When agencies consider implementing evidence-based practice, there is a temptation to find shortcuts and strategies to cut costs. For some aspects of some programs, this may be possible. Unfortunately, the jury is still out regarding many of these factors, especially when there is uncertainty about the essential elements and activities in the practice model's theory of change, and to what extent flexibility in their delivery is possible. Studies such as Smith-Boydston et al. (2014) demonstrate the importance of assessing the impacts of such decisions. In that case, the youth and community no longer received the promised benefit from MST service delivery because they were no longer receiving MST.

Fidelity monitoring can be challenging in real-world settings, leading some to question how realistic it is for agencies to routinely measure adherence to a practice model's elements and activities. This challenge may be due to the fact that many fidelity monitoring strategies were developed primarily as a means to establish internal validity for efficacy or effectiveness trials. Many of these approaches are labor intensive, involving video or audiotape review and expert feedback. Much work remains to develop effective fidelity monitoring approaches that are pragmatic and feasible in community-based settings. Furthermore, a majority of practices have not validated their fidelity tools, nor developed clear and simple benchmarks that indicate the practice is being delivered with fidelity. These limitations and challenges must be addressed in the coming years, especially as organizations are increasingly required by funding sources to demonstrate effective delivery of evidence-based practices with fidelity.

Can simple outcome monitoring be a complimentary strategy, or perhaps even an alternative strategy to fidelity monitoring? Fidelity monitoring was developed as a necessary implementation driver for achieving improved client outcomes. If a client is not achieving improved outcomes, then perhaps that is when fidelity to the practice model should be evaluated. Thus, for clients achieving improved outcomes, spending time and resources on fidelity monitoring may not be necessary. Outcome monitoring is an essential part of good service delivery and can be monitored by using standardized measures or individualized progress measures. Interestingly, a recent study found that while monitoring fidelity and outcomes are acceptable to practitioners, there was a strong preference for individualized progress measures (Cook, Hausman, Jensen-Doss, & Hawkey, 2017).

Practical Challenges During Initial Implementation

The stage of initial implementation is one of "high risk and high gain." In many ways, this is where the rubber meets the road and agencies learn if their preparation to implement the new practice was sufficient. In an ideal world, after a thorough preparation of the organization during the installation stage and addressing implementation challenges in a transformation zone, staff are eager and ready to deliver the new practice, referral pathways are identified and established, and clients receive the benefits of the intervention right away. However, the organization and community context are often in flux and it is not uncommon to hear statements like this during initial implementation of a new practice model:

1. **"I don't know what I'm doing."**

What might contribute to a statement like this from a newly trained practitioner, supervisor, or manager? Perhaps they did not receive adequate training prior to initiating the new practice. Even if there was adequate training, uncertainty or low confidence is not unusual. However, there may also be organizational policy or procedure that makes delivery of the new practice feel chaotic and disorganized.

It is important to consider organizational factors that may be contributing to such a statement and not simply assume the problem is in the person expressing confusion. Encouraging free expression of such sentiment and then exploring with those who share it can clarify the source of this concern. Statements such as this are cause to pause and consider the thoroughness of installation stage activities.

2. **"There aren't enough clients eligible for the new practice."**

Statements such as this suggest a couple of implementation challenges. Clients who can benefit from the new practice may not be available because the community is unaware or does not understand how the new practice could be helpful for clients. If this is the case, the implementation driver of systems-level interventions requires attention. Administrators and managers should engage key stakeholders to ensure they understand and appreciate the value of the new practice. Any confusion or needed clarification about how to refer clients to the service can be addressed.

Occasionally, there may be sufficient client referrals but they do not represent the population targeted by the new practice. In this situation, those making such referrals are disappointed or frustrated when their client is denied service. Administrators and managers must communicate clear inclusionary and exclusionary criteria to stakeholders and explain the rationale for any exceptions. When denying service, it is helpful to follow-up directly with stakeholders to explain why the client was not eligible for treatment and to clarify client criteria for the new practice. If possible, troubleshooting a more appropriate referral can create goodwill with the referral source.

Not having enough clients to benefit from the new practice may also indicate a breakdown of communication or a misunderstanding within the organization. This often occurs when intake assessments and direct services are provided by different people. During installation of the new practice, *all staff including administrative support staff* should receive training on client characteristics, the elements and activities of the new practice, and how this produces improved outcomes (theory of change). This orientation should be followed by monitoring numbers and types of referrals. Patterns of appropriate referral should be highlighted and receive positive reinforcement, while those making inappropriate referrals should be reminded and coached. The entire organization must engage in new behavior pertinent to the new practice.

3. **"My first client completed only two sessions. My second client keeps no-showing. This is not working."**

These statements are not uncommon from newly trained practitioners. Frequently, the first few cases do not go as expected or planned. In coaching, it is important to acknowledge that this is part of both the individual and the organizational learning process. It is especially common for the first few sessions to be delivered "mechanistically"—that is, the practitioner may be overly focused on getting through the activities and elements of the new practice, and not yet be able to smoothly nor fully integrate them with their experience and existing skills. This is the space where "art meets science." It takes quite a bit of confidence to merge knowledge or skills developed in training, or knowledge derived from reading practice protocol, and blend this with "nonspecific" elements such as displaying warmth, and empathy, authenticity, active listening that validates the client's experience. Such confidence develops over time with good coaching, and this should be emphasized.

There is a phenomenon that implementation scientists refer to as "Type III error." That is failure to implement the new practice as planned. This is particularly likely during the stage of initial implementation. It may be important to plan and predict, to normalize this experience with staff during the initial training events as well as in coaching and consultation. They must not feel they have failed clients. Instead, the organization will become more productive by encouraging active problem-solving, identifying what went wrong, and developing plans to remedy it with the next visit or the next client.

4. **"There is no way this practice can be delivered to *my* clients in the way it is described in the manual."**

This forceful sentiment is often heard during initial training events and during post-training consultation or coaching. An important first step in addressing such sentiment is to clarify the primary concerns. For example, sentiments such as this may emanate from an impression that the new practice is not sufficient for the levels of behavioral severity displayed by clients. This is often a side effect of using simplistic examples during training in well-meaning but shortsighted attempts to create early confidence in an adequate demonstration of knowledge and skill.

Such forceful sentiments may also cover concerns about cultural appropriateness and how clients may experience the new practice. These sentiments may cover differences in theoretical orientation and belief about what causes and maintains behavior, or perhaps a deep belief that the current and more accustomed approach is the most valid for clients. The latter point may even be a product from a training environment that communicated, albeit unintentionally, that the reason for the new practice is because the current and accustomed practice is ineffective. It is important to anticipate this perception. Trainers must consciously present new information in a way that increases receptivity and decreases defensiveness.

There is rarely "one right answer." The best strategy is to ask questions to elicit and validate a practitioner's, supervisor's or manager's perspective while clarifying any information that could be helpful to identify and work through their concerns. To work through strong sentiments about a new evidence-based practice, it may be helpful to review in advance and to be well-versed in chapter four's presentation of evidence-based practice myths, misconceptions, and facts. These myths and misconceptions are not uncommon and may comprise some of the basis for such forceful sentiment.

5. **"I'm not getting evaluated on my delivery of the new practice and I'm not getting paid more, so is this really worth the extra time and trouble?"**

These types of statements or reactions suggest limitations in the installation of a new practice. They are always a cause to pause and carefully consider the organization's introduction and installation of the new practice. What are the personal benefits of delivering the new practice and what are the consequences of not doing so? Did the organization engage staff sufficiently to address these concerns? Often training efforts focus on client benefits, but most staff believe that they are already doing good work. Therefore, focusing exclusively on client benefits may not be a strong enough incentive for staff to make the effort and work through challenges associated with learning to implement a new practice.

Formal incentives such as increased pay for delivery of evidence-based practice are a potentially impactful strategy. Of course, many factors determine whether this is feasible, especially considering the historically low reimbursement rates from Medicaid and insurance that drive much of an agency's business model. Nevertheless, building effective delivery of the new practice into incentives such as annual salary merit increases may be a potent strategy. On the other side of contingency reinforcement, some agencies require staff to sign contracts prior to training that obligate them to repay the cost of training and materials if they do not deliver the new practice or if they leave the agency within a specified time period. To our knowledge, there is no research indicating the effectiveness of that approach in driving behavior change.

6. **"I'll be evaluated on delivery of the new practice, and I'm anxious."**

Anxiety is normal when enacting a new practice or behavior. It is potentially compounded when evaluative criteria are in play. Agencies must have a supportive infrastructure and culture that provides time and space to learn while simultaneously holding staff accountable for effective delivery of the new practice with fidelity.

This can be a delicate line to walk. Agency administrators may want to consider strategies such as temporary reductions in productivity requirements to allow for additional time for staff to focus on learning the new model and to participate in model-pertinent coaching or consultation. Early evaluations should have a developmental focus and help the practitioner identify areas to focus on for growth. Personalized goal setting, with support and monitoring by a trusted supervisor or consultant, can be effective in improving delivery of the new practice while building a staff confidence and ability to influence their learning process.

Summary

This is not an exhaustive list of potential initial implementation stage challenges. In addition to these more common experiences, each setting has its unique set of expected and unexpected challenges. This is why it is important to begin small, to identify a zone of transformation in the agency where these experiences and challenges can be more easily addressed before scaling up the new practice throughout the organization (Bertram, Blase, & Fixsen, 2015). As mentioned in the previous chapter, Powell et al. (2015) compiled a comprehensive list of 73 implementation strategies that provide conceptual guidance for agencies to consider supports that may need to be in place or adjusted during initial implementation of a new practice.

References

Beidas, R. S., Barmish, A. J., & Kendall, P. C. (2009). Training as usual: Can therapist behavior change after reading a manual and attending a brief workshop on cognitive behavioral therapy for youth anxiety? *Behavior Therapist, 32*(5), 97–101.

Bertram, R. M., Blase, K. A., & Fixsen, D. L. (2015). Improving programs and outcomes: Implementation frameworks and organization change. *Research on Social Work Practice, 25*(4), 477–487.

Carroll, C., Patterson, M., Wood, S., Booth, A., Rick, J., & Balain, S. (2007). A conceptual framework for implementation fidelity. *Implementation Science, 2*(1), 40.

Cook, J. R., Hausman, E. M., Jensen-Doss, A., & Hawley, K. M. (2017). Assessment practices of child clinicians: Results from a national survey. *Assessment, 24*(2), 210–221.

Crane, R. S., Kuyken, W., Williams, J. M. G., Hastings, R. P., Cooper, L., & Fennell, M. J. (2012). Competence in teaching mindfulness-based courses: concepts, development and assessment. *Mindfulness, 3*(1), 76–84.

Dorsey, S., Pullmann, M. D., Deblinger, E., Berliner, L., Kerns, S. E., Thompson, K., … & Garland, A. F. (2013). Improving practice in community-based settings: A randomized trial of supervision—study protocol. *Implementation Science, 8*(1), 89.

Hawkins, J. D., Catalano, R. F., & Kuklinski, M. R. (2014). Communities that care. In *Encyclopedia of criminology and criminal justice* (pp. 393–408). New York, NY: Springer.

Julian, D. A. (2006). A community practice model for community psychologists and some examples of the application of community practice skills from the partnerships for success initiative in Ohio. *American Journal of Community Psychology, 37*(1–2), 21–27.

Kerns, S. E. U., McCormick, E., Negrete, A., Carey, C., Haaland, W., & Waller, S. (2017). Predicting post-training implementation of a parenting intervention. *Journal of Children's Services, 12*(4), 302–315.

Lyon, A. R., Stirman, S. W., Kerns, S. E. U., & Bruns, E. J. (2011). Developing the mental health workforce: Review and application of training approaches from multiple disciplines. *Administration and Policy in Mental Health and Mental Health Services Research, 38*(4), 238–253.

Powell, B. J., Waltz, T. J., Chinman, M. J., Damschroder, L. J., Smith, J. L., Matthieu, M. M., … & Kirchner, J. E. (2015). A refined compilation of implementation strategies: Results from the Expert Recommendations for Implementing Change (ERIC) project. *Implementation Science, 10*(1), 21.

Schoenwald, S. K., Sheidow, A. J., & Letourneau, E. J. (2004). Toward effective quality assurance in evidence-based practice: Links between expert consultation, therapist fidelity, and child outcomes. *Journal of Clinical Child and Adolescent Psychology, 33*(1), 94–104.

Smith-Boydston, J. M., Holtzman, R. J., & Roberts, M. C. (2014). Transportability of multisystemic therapy to community settings: Can a program sustain outcomes without MST services oversight? *Child & Youth Care Forum, 43*(5), 593–605.

Tan, K. M. (2002). Influence of educational outreach visits on behavioral change in health professionals. *Journal of Continuing Education in the Health Professions, 22*(2), 122–124.

Wandersman, A., Imm, P., Chinman, M., & Kaftarian, S. (2000). Getting to outcomes: A results-based approach to accountability. *Evaluation and Program Planning, 23*(3), 389–395.

Chapter 10
Troubleshooting Implementation Challenges

Have you ever bought something online but when it arrives, it does not seem to be what you expected? Sometimes implementation of evidence-based practice can be similar. Reality can be a bit different than what we expected. A well-planned installation of an evidence-based practice that begins initial implementation in a transformation zone will mitigate many of the most substantial problems. This chapter anticipates the most common challenges and suggests strategies to address them. This is not an exhaustive review. As in life, there are those things you can anticipate and those you cannot.

Installation and Sustainability Expenses

Careful selection, installation, and initial implementation activities support sustainability. However, installation and sustaining activities supporting evidence-based practices are often more expensive than "continuing treatment as usual," and the cost is a primary concern of organizations seeking to adopt new practices (e.g., Proctor et al., 2011; Wisdom, Chor, Hoagwood, & Horwitz, 2014). What contributes to the greater expense?

Most evidence-based practices require a rigorous training process. Contracts with treatment experts to provide well-developed and tested training processes are an obvious expense. As seen in Chap. 6, testing an innovative practice to identify its efficacy and effectiveness, then making adaptations in dissemination studies require a significant investment of time and resources, and not all innovative practices receive full grant support.

In addition, while staff participate in installation activities as well as in later training and coaching processes, they are not engaging clients in a billable or reimbursable service. As discussed in Chaps. 8 and 9, during initial implementation, the organization should start small with select staff in a zone of transformation. This limits the investment of resources, while the organization addresses and learns from initial implementation challenges. However, those selected staff usually have reduced

© Springer Nature Switzerland AG 2019
R. Bertram and S. Kerns, *Selecting and Implementing Evidence-Based Practice*,
https://doi.org/10.1007/978-3-030-11325-4_10

caseloads to allow for adequate preparation and coaching with consultants. Though this initially constrains revenue, starting small facilitates more manageable individual and organizational learning for subsequent scaling up of the new practice across the agency. If allowed by the program developer, staff initially trained and coached in the transformation zone may become trainers and coaches to other staff in that scaling up process.

As this scaling up process unfolds, there can be specific resources that must be purchased such as workbooks, manuals, equipment, or special toys and games necessary for effective delivery of the new practice. Additional expenses also may include the revision of marketing materials, meetings with agency partners to ensure they understand the new practice and criteria for client referral, as well as staff incentives for participation. Long-term implementation efforts require some resources to train new therapists over time to account for turnover in staff.

The extent to which these costs are incremental over "treatment as usual" still needs to be confirmed. An initial attempt to study this found that for general outpatient services (i.e., programs that deliver service during weekly in-office sessions), the incremental costs averaged approximately $114 per client. More intensive practices like MST require multiple visits per week, in the family home, at the school or in the community (thus requiring practitioner transportation). For MST, the incremental costs averaged substantially more, at $1548 per client (Kerns, Levin, Leith, Carey, & Uomoto, 2016).

However, when examined through the lens of community impact, evidence-based practices often save money. This is particularly true for practices that focus on preventing or reducing high-cost deleterious outcomes such as out-of-home placements, criminal recidivism, and inpatient hospitalization. For example, in a two-year period, Dopp et al. (2018) identified taxpayer savings of $34,326 per youth served through Multisystemic Therapy.

The Washington State Institute for Public Policy (WSIPP) is one of the most highly regarded entities documenting the cost-benefit of evidence-based practices. Astute readers will recall that this institute was influential in clarifying criteria to define the extent of evidence supporting innovative practices. Their website (www.wsipp.wa.gov) listed in the appendix at the conclusion of this book is exceptionally useful for both academic and behavioral healthcare programs.

In 2017, WSIPP conducted cost-benefit analyses for 28 evidence-based practices in mental health services. Nineteen practices had favorable cost-benefit ratios ranging from a savings of $552 to over $21,000. For the other nine practices, costs were more substantial than the benefits (Washington State Institute for Public Policy, 2017). However, it is important to note that these benefits are most substantially realized within the justice system and education system, or systems that address victim rights or access to Medicaid, managed care, and social security. In these systems, organizations may "foot the bill," but not be the direct beneficiaries of these savings.

Some research indicates that the implementation of evidence-based practices can produce cost benefits within the organization. For example, clients may be less likely to skip appointments, while well-supported staff are less likely to quit their jobs, thus reducing costs associated with low productivity and turnover (e.g., Aarons, Sommerfeld, Hecht, Silovsky, & Chaffin, 2009). When reimbursement rates are commensurate with additional costs, financial barriers can be mitigated. This often requires administrative advocacy at the local and state levels, especially if the primary funder is Medicaid.

In the Kerns et al. (2016) cost study, approximately half of the agencies experienced some financial benefits from the implementation of evidence-based practice, but there was substantial cost variability across agencies. Agency-specific cost containment strategies, combined with leveraging the principle of economy of scale, accounted for much of the cost variability. Programs that were operating at full capacity had much lower costs per client than those who were struggling with aspects of implementation (Kerns et al., 2016).

Let's examine Multisystemic Therapy (MST) as an example of the economy of scale principle. One MST team includes from two to four practitioners plus one half-time supervisor. The practitioners engage from four to six families at a time, and the average length of treatment is about 4 months. Therefore, a practitioner can realistically engage between 12 and 18 families per year. There are several non-negotiable costs associated with implementing MST that include required days of training for practitioners and supervisors, fidelity and outcome data collection and monitoring, booster training, and other activities that support maintaining the organization's recognition as a licensed MST provider.

Let's assume that these overall, non-negotiable and implementation costs (not including staff salaries, labor, and other overhead costs) are about $30,000 per year (note, this is not a precisely accurate number, we are using this number here for illustrative purposes only). This portion of the cost is for training, consultation, and implementation supports. If an organization maintains a team of 2 practitioners, each with a caseload of 4 clients, the cost per client family is $1250 ($30,000/12 families) x (2 practitioners) = $1250. If an organization maintains a team of 4 practitioners, each with a steady caseload of 6 clients, the cost is $416 per client family ($30,000/(18 families) x (4 practitioners) = $416). This is a threefold difference in cost per client family based on the non-negotiable implementation costs.

Of course, this analysis does not include variable costs such as staff salaries, which would be higher in the second example. But it does illustrate the power of economy of scale. Frequently, when an agency is struggling financially to support an evidence-based practice, there are implementation-related solutions that can help reduce or resolve funding challenges. For example, as discussed in Chap. 9, the administration can carefully examine, clarify, and strengthen referral pathways to ensure practitioners provide service to the maximum number of clients appropriate for the intervention. Also reviewed in Chap. 9, careful attention to implementation drivers by administrators and managers can reduce staff turn-over. However, monitoring implementation drivers is dependent upon adjusting data systems to support implementation decisions. We'll more closely examine this key implementation driver in Chap. 11.

Limited Support from Management

Sometimes selection of a new practice begins with practitioners who initiate exploration and learning about a new evidence-based practice. They may convince their immediate managers or supervisors of the merits of adopting the new practice. However, sometimes the "top brass" are not convinced. They may be conceptually supportive of the idea, but lack the passion required for successful implementation. In these situations, sometimes supervisors experience a squeeze between upper management and practitioners—they are not the ones to directly deliver the intervention, yet they are tasked with supervising its implementation.

Unfortunately, the role of administrators or managers is amongst the least studied in evidence-based practice implementation. Greg Aarons and colleagues discussed a phase-based model for implementation. Their phases include exploration, preparation, implementation, and sustainment (EPIS), and they described the role of leadership as being most prominent in the preparation and implementation phases (Aarons et al., 2016). However, in a review of rigorous evaluations of different implementation factors, only five studies specifically examined leadership, with only one doing so using a randomized control design (Novins et al., 2013).

Furthermore, in most organizations, upper administrative positions are responsible for a range of different programs and practices. The addition of a new evidence-based practice model in one of the programs may represent a very small proportion of the agency's overall services for which they are responsible. Nevertheless, insufficient monitoring of the newly introduced practice by administrators is a certain recipe for its ineffective implementation. Thus, when the impetus to adopt an evidence-based practice emerges from practitioners, it is essential that strategies engage administrators early and often throughout installation and initial implementation stages. Administrators must align policy, procedure, and data systems, staff selection criteria and processes to support the new practice. They have unique access to funding sources, policy makers, and community leaders that is necessary to market and sustain the new evidence-based practice.

Adaptive administrators negotiate these many responsibilities through implementation teams. Ideally, these teams are formed in the exploration and installation stages of implementation and include a stratified sample of staff, as well as key community partners, and expert consultants. Implementation teams problem-solve initial implementation challenges in the transformation zone, and lessons learned guide administrators as they plan to scale the practice throughout the program or organization (Bertram, Blase, & Fixsen, 2015; Bertram, Blase, Shern, Shea, & Fixsen, 2011).

Integrating or Adding

When organizations fail to adjust implementation drivers, when they simply "train and hope," staff experience the new practice as an additional responsibility. Quite frankly, they have usually experienced this with the introduction of previous new practices. In such situations, it is not unusual to hear staff say that "this too shall soon pass."

Careful attention to installation and initial implementation stage activities aligns agency infrastructure (implementation drivers) with the new practice. This alignment of infrastructure integrates rather than adding the new practice into the organization. Well-aligned implementation drivers develop and support staff competence and confidence in the delivery of the new practice, a clear signal that "this will not soon pass." With careful attention to exploration and adoption, installation and initial implementation stage activities, an organization can achieve fidelity and outcome benchmarks in from two to four years (Bertram et al., 2015). Achieving these benchmarks is evidence that the new practice is well integrated and sustainable.

As the new practice is scaled up from a transformation zone across the organization, practitioners and supervisors will have some cases in which treatment began prior to adoption and installation of the new practice. During initial implementation, staff expend substantially more time and energy developing competence and confidence in the new practice while still addressing older cases. The challenge of balancing this workload should be predicted, normalized, and validated.

Implementation is a process, not an event. As implementation drivers are adjusted and data emerge that support coaching toward greater effectiveness and delivering the new practice with fidelity, the organization will experience a transition. It will become clear that the new practice is fully incorporated within a supportive agency infrastructure. Questions and debates about the longevity of the new practice diminish as more and more client cases (eventually including even the older ones) are engaged in the new practice. As full implementation is achieved, there are clear and reliable strategies ensuring appropriate referrals. Practitioners, supervisors, and managers know what is expected and can fulfill these responsibilities with increasing confidence and competence. Fidelity and client outcome data provide evidence of this, and that implementation drivers are well aligned, supporting staff in effectively fulfilling these responsibilities.

However, some organizations stall in the process of initial implementation. This often occurs when transformation zones and implementation teams are not used, resulting in the organization "biting off more than it can chew." When this occurs, the organization becomes consumed by long and not well-coordinated periods of problem-solving. Lengthy start-up periods are disheartening, stressful, and contribute to burn-out and resignations. When you hear practitioners repeatedly saying things like "we're still building this airplane while we try our best to fly it" or, less colorfully, "we're still working out the kinks," this is cause to pause. The organization must closely examine what it has or has not done to integrate the new practice into its infrastructure. The following is a non-exhaustive list of considerations that may be useful to consider:

- Do staff understand the intended purpose of the new evidence-based practice?

- How well do staff understand its elements and activities and how the new practice improves client outcomes?

- Has the organization created time and space in the program and in caseload assignments so that staff develop competence and confidence in delivering the new practice?

- Are agency partners well informed and are structures in place to support appropriate client referrals? If intake staff are used, do they have proper training and receive feedback for appropriate client referral?

- Are staff selection criteria and processes aligned with the new practice? Do new hire training and coaching processes and initial case assignments support efficient and effective uptake of knowledge and skill development?

- Are materials needed to deliver the new practice always readily and easily available?

- Does case documentation inform coaching and supervision of the new practice?

- Are scheduling structures and processes aligned with the activities and elements of the new practice? Does this include scheduling fidelity supports such as coaching and case consultation calls?

- Is it clear how the implementation of the new practice is related to staff evaluation? Is this reasonable? How can fidelity and improved outcomes be meaningfully acknowledged and rewarded?

- Are there hidden disincentives for delivering the new practice? Does a focus on productivity clash with necessary elements of the new practice such as phone calls and visits to engage school personnel or natural supports from the community?

Organizations experiencing a lengthy initial implementation can identify staff who appear to be understanding and implementing the new practice with confidence and competence. This identification should not be anecdotal. Case documentation, fidelity, and client outcome data provide the best guide in a search for these staff. Once identified, they should be engaged in a practical and specific discussion about what they do that works well and what supports them. What works and what does not? What could be done differently? This discussion will be far more productive if it focuses through the components of the new practice and upon alignment of implementation drivers.

Staff Resistance

When not identified and addressed early staff resistance to a new practice, can have a toxic effect on its initial implementation and uptake at an agency. Sources of this challenge are multifaceted. If the organization has recently implemented other practices, or is currently implementing several new practices, resistance may be a symptom of "change fatigue."

Sometimes there is an organizational history of introducing a new practice and when its implementation stalls, another practice is introduced. In this context, staff understandably may anticipate a short life expectancy for the new practice. As a result, their investment of time, effort, and energy in the new practice may be limited as they await its eventual demise. This phenomenon can be so common staff refer to the new practice as a "helicopter model." It arrives with a flurry, stays a short time, and then departs in the flurry of the arrival of another practice.

Often not considered, for some staff, new practices may be perceived as a personal affront. Because the organization is changing the practice model, these staff may feel that the agency did not value their prior work. Because they feel confident and independent in their previous responsibilities, they may experience necessary coaching and fidelity monitoring in the new practice as an invalidating backward step. This new oversight may be viewed as micromanaging at best, stifling, restrictive, and punitive at worst.

There are many studies (e.g., Aarons & Sawitzky, 2006; Kerns et al., 2017) that demonstrate the predictive nature of attitudes about evidence-based interventions on implementation. Those with more favorable attitudes are more likely to readily adopt a new evidence-based practice. Those with less favorable attitudes are less likely to adopt the new practice. This is another reason why transformation of academic curricula is so important.

However, most studies fail to demonstrate movement or change of attitude during implementation. Attitudes or beliefs are critical constructs that should be assessed during installation and initial implementation of a new practice. Staff selection processes and criteria should identify those with favorable attitudes about evidence-based practice, about supervision, and about using data to coach them toward greater competence and confidence. By baselining attitudes and beliefs in the staff selection process, after a period of training, coaching and use of data in delivery of the practice, the organization can again assess staff attitudes and beliefs. These results can serve as an organizational fidelity measure, informing the agency how well its realignment of implementation drivers is developing staff competence and confidence.

Whether introducing an evidence-based practice to current staff or to potential new-hires, how the agency presents the opportunities of the new practice will have a significant impact. Organization leadership that selects new practices behind closed doors will have a steeper hill to climb toward understanding and acceptance. Transparently engaging staff and community partners in the process of exploration and adoption of evidence-based practices takes time and effort but will produce greater understanding and investment in the new practice. This was recently done across the state of Missouri to initiate selection of new child welfare philosophy and practice. The process of seven community conversations generated significant staff enthusiasm and began to reposition Missouri Children's Division with its community partners (Bertram, Decker, Gillies, & Choi, 2017).

The role of organization culture and climate is well established. As Peter Drucker famously quipped, "culture eats strategy for lunch" (Eaton, 2015). How staff and community partners are engaged in exploration and adoption of a new practice, the careful alignment of implementation drivers during its installation, and reviewing model-pertinent data to adjust these drivers and processes during initial implementation improves organizational climate and culture. When infrastructure (implementation drivers) is not well aligned with delivery of the practice model, agency culture adversely impacts climate with consequent negative impact on fidelity and outcomes (Aarons et al., 2016).

Client Engagement and Motivation

Let's shift our lens to client experience during initial implementation. We've reviewed how practitioners learning a new practice, especially if it is their first time learning an evidence-based practice, do not feel competent or confident. Initially, staff focus more upon structures and content of the new practice's elements and activities. This may compromise their ability to fully engage clients in the treatment process.

Clients can perceive this and may experience doubts about the service. They may withdraw from treatment, participate sporadically, and like the practitioner, may not fully engage in the treatment process. These situations pose risk for clients, practitioners, and the organization. Clients may not receive the intended treatment and may not achieve desired outcomes. Practitioners may decide that the new practice is unacceptable to clients or too difficult for them to deliver. The organization can then experience diminished billable units of service, low staff morale, and even resignations.

If data demonstrate that clients are sporadically withdrawing from service, if planned reports on the focus of coaching identify this challenge, or if practitioners' confidence and morale seem lower, managers, supervisors, or coaches can engage practitioners in a "Plan and Predict" discussion prior to seeing their clients. Ideally, this should occur prior to initial contact with the client, but this can also work retroactively. Here is a sample idea to prompt discussion:

Predict. *When learning a new model, it can be difficult to hold all the details of the new program in your head while delivering the session content in a natural and authentic way. That's totally normal. Sometimes, because of this, it means that your first few clients miss sessions or that their participation and motivation is not strong. Do you remember when you first started working as a clinician? You made it through those first few sessions and you can count on being able to do the same here.*

Plan. *What can I do to help when you worry that you're not effective in session?*

The practitioner may or may not be able to identify specific help needed. The supervisor should be prepared to coach the practitioner to identify abilities developed before the new practice model was introduced, then walk through to apply those abilities in the elements or activity of the new practice.

It may also be valuable to consider how to promote practitioner practice of the model outside of a formal client session. This is commonly done in role play in individual supervision or in coached learning groups. As discussed in Chap. 8, behavioral rehearsal is a potent tool to help practitioners build mastery. It provides staff opportunity to gain familiarity with the elements and activities of a practice model while finding an authentic voice that integrates their previous abilities.

Cultural Relevance

Cultural relevance of a practice can present an implementation challenge for the organization. Evidence-based practices usually begin in a specific region with its particular composition of cultures and demographics (recall the efficacy, effectiveness, and dissemination studies in Chap. 6). Although interventions are largely tested in geographically specific areas, research suggests that EBPs can still have validity in diverse settings (Castro, Barrera, & Holleran Steiker, 2010). However, some accommodations may be necessary to increase the relevancy of the intervention for a specific area, culture, or client population (Chu, Leino, Pflum, & Sue, 2016).

> *Language shapes our thoughts, so let's anticipate and avoid confusion that might arise from what seem to be nearly synonymous words. What is the difference between "accommodation" and "modification?" Take a moment and write your definition without using a dictionary app. Then continue reading about the critical difference of these terms in addressing implementation challenges of evidence-based practices.*

Accommodations do not change the core elements and activities of the practice model. Recall our discussion in Chap. 8 about a practice model's "adaptable periphery." Accommodations such as using local examples or folklore to explain a concept, or using language specific to a region or group can address cultural relevance implementation challenges. Making accommodations to a practice model might include providing supports for attending group sessions aligned with local customs and culture such as providing dinner. These adaptations enhance cultural relevance.

Modifications are more substantial and can potentially impact the core components of the practice model. For example, if cognitive concepts are the key elements of an evidence-based model, and if the practice activities present them in a linear fashion, this might be an implementation challenge when engaging clients from cultures that have a more circular or integrated way of thinking. Modifications are deeper changes in the tested activities and elements of an evidence-based practice model. They require careful thought, engaging a researcher or purveyor to ensure that such changes do not have a substantial impact on the effectiveness of the practice.

It bears mention that practitioners are sometimes more skeptical about the cultural relevance of a program than the clients themselves. For example, an interesting study by Morawska et al. (2011) and a follow-up Moraska et al. study in 2012, revealed that parents from a variety of diverse backgrounds rated parenting strategies and skills that were part of an evidence-based intervention as much more acceptable than practitioners thought they would. This finding suggests that it may be helpful to first try the new practice as it was originally designed.

Organizations can anticipate cultural relevance implementation challenges as they install these data systems. This could include a cultural relevance monthly report that simply presented participation patterns of clients by age, gender, race, ethnicity, and culture. By reviewing these reports and comparing them with fidelity and outcome data, the organization can determine whether modification of a key element or activity may be necessary. If so, then prospective problem solving by the organization with the practice model purveyor will be important. Practitioners should not make modifications prior to this consultation to ascertain the potential impact of such changes!

Managing Expectations

When new practices are initiated, the excitement and enthusiasm can foster unrealistic expectations. High hopes without diligent and effective implementation leave organizations, staff, and the community vulnerable to disappointment. It is critical to be realistic about improving client outcomes. It takes time during installation stage activities to align implementation drivers with the evidence-based practice. During initial implementation in a transformation zone, these drivers may be further adjusted until practitioners begin to achieve fidelity and client outcome expectations. Then the practice can be scaled up across the organization. However, funding concerns or wanting to build upon staff excitement may lead an organization to scale up initial implementation of the practice before fidelity and outcome data signal implementation readiness. This is when unexpected implementation challenges may emerge.

This chapter identified some common challenges that emerge during initial implementation of evidence-based practice, as well as strategies to anticipate and address them. It is unlikely an organization would encounter *all* of these challenges, and just as unlikely that they would not encounter *any* of them. Focusing through implementation frameworks to guide program selection and installation helps mitigate these challenges.

> *When discussion of a challenge focuses upon individual persons or personality characteristics, this is often a caution flag warning us to first examine how well implementation stage activities and alignment of implementation drivers have been enacted.*

Starting small in transformation zones makes implementation challenges more manageable. Use of well-composed implementation teams that focus upon alignment of implementation drivers and that are informed by model pertinent data can address most challenges. If that team has adaptive leadership and a spirit of problem-solving through collaboration, if it is willing to be creative, there are few challenges that are truly insurmountable.

Summary

It is impossible to provide an exhaustive list of all challenges that may be faced during implementation. However, it is helpful to consider likely challenges and do active problem-solving ahead of time. This may prevent the challenge from occurring and may help design strategies to effectively manage the challenge should it emerge. In addition, establishing a transformation zone and a well-composed implementation team is instrumental to effectively and efficiently address implementation challenges.

References

Aarons, G. A., Green, A. E., Trott, E., Willging, C. E., Torres, E. M., Ehrhart, M. G., & Roesch, S. C. (2016). The roles of system and organizational leadership in system-wide evidence-based intervention sustainment: A mixed-method study. *Administration and Policy in Mental Health and Mental Health Services Research, 43*(6), 991–1008

Aarons, G. A., & Sawitzky, A. C. (2006). Organizational culture and climate and mental health provider attitudes toward evidence-based practice. *Psychological Services, 3*(1), 61.

Aarons, G. A., Sommerfeld, D., Hecht, D., Silovsky, J., & Chaffin, M. (2009). The impact of evidence-based practice implementation and fidelity monitoring on staff turnover: Evidence for a protective effect. *Journal of Consulting and Clinical Psychology, 77*(2), 270–280.

Bertram, R. M., Blase, K. A., & Fixsen, D. L. (2015). Improving programs and outcomes: Implementation frameworks and organization change. *Research on Social Work Practice, 25*(4), 477–487.

Bertram, R., Blase, K., Shern, D., Shea, P., & Fixsen, D. (2011). *Policy research brief: Implementation opportunities and challenges for prevention and promotion initiatives.* Alexandria, VA: National Association of State Mental Health Program Directors (NASMHPD).

Bertram, R. M., Decker, T., Gillies, M. E., & Choi, S. W. (2017). Transforming Missouri's child welfare system: Community conversations, organizational assessment, and university partnership. *Families in Society: The Journal of Contemporary Social Services, 98*(1), 9–17.

Castro, F. G., Barrera, M., Jr., & Holleran Steiker, L. K. (2010). Issues and challenges in the design of culturally adapted evidence-based interventions. *Annual Review of Clinical Psychology, 6,* 213–239.

Chu, J., Leino, A., Pflum, S., & Sue, S. (2016). A model for the theoretical basis of cultural competency to guide psychotherapy. *Professional Psychology: Research and Practice, 47*(1), 18.

Dopp, A. R., Coen, A. S., Smith, A. B., Reno, J., Bernstein, D. H., Kerns, S. E. U., et al. (2018). Economic impact of the statewide implementation of an evidence-based treatment: Multisystemic therapy in New Mexico. *Behavior Therapy, 49*(4), 551–566.

Eaton, D. (2015). Making the shift: Leading first with who we are, not what we do. *People and Strategy, 38*(3), 46.

Kerns, S. E. U., Levin, C., Leith, J., Carey, C., & Uomoto, A. (2016). *Preliminary estimate of costs associated with implementing research and evidence-based practices for children and youth in Washington State (Report).* University of Washington School of Medicine, Division of Public Behavioral Health and Justice Policy. Retrieved from https://www.hca.wa.gov/assets/program/ebt-cost-study-report.pdf.

Kerns, S. E. U., McCormick, E., Negrete, A., Carey, C., Haaland, W., & Waller, S. (2017). Predicting post-training implementation of a parenting intervention. *Journal of Children's Services, 12*(4), 302–315.

Morawska, A., Sanders, M., Goadby, E., Headley, C., Hodge, L., McAuliffe, C., ... & Anderson, E. (2011). Is the Triple P-Positive Parenting Program acceptable to parents from culturally diverse backgrounds? *Journal of Child and Family Studies, 20*(5), 614–622.

Morawska, A., Sanders, M. R., O'Brien, J., McAuliffe, C., Pope, S., & Anderson, E. (2012). Practitioner perceptions of the use of the Triple P–Positive Parenting Program with families from culturally diverse backgrounds. *Australian Journal of Primary Health, 18*(4), 313–320.

Novins, D. K., Green, A. E., Legha, R. K., & Aarons, G. A. (2013). Dissemination and implementation of evidence-based practices for child and adolescent mental health: A systematic review. *Journal of the American Academy of Child and Adolescent Psychiatry, 52*(10), 1009–1025.

Proctor, E., Silmere, H., Raghavan, R., Hovmand, P., Aarons, G., Bunger, A., ... & Hensley, M. (2011). Outcomes for implementation research: Conceptual distinctions, measurement challenges, and research agenda. *Administration and Policy in Mental Health and Mental Health Services Research, 38*(2), 65–76.

Wisdom, J. P., Chor, K. H. B., Hoagwood, K. E., & Horwitz, S. M. (2014). Innovation adoption: A review of theories and constructs. *Administration and Policy in Mental Health and Mental Health Services Research, 41*(4), 480–502.

Chapter 11
Data-Informed Implementation

Well-organized implementation planning processes use data to provide accountability within an organization as well as between the organization, the community, and funding sources. Being "data-informed" or using "data-driven decision making" are frequently used terms, in implementation science and frameworks. This chapter expands upon discussions in previous chapters about implementation data. First, we discuss a few practical examples of how asking the right questions and developing useful plans and data to address them can inform the selection and adoption of an evidence-based practice to address particular community concerns. We present a specific example of how Partnerships for Success, a model for conducting this process was applied in a Pacific Northwest community.

This chapter also addresses the establishment of implementation data feedback loops during installation stage activities, and during actual implementation, the use of symptom monitoring data systems including lower-cost approaches such as the EBP toolkit and PracticeWise clinical dashboard. We conclude with an example of how data inform implementation of Multisystemic Therapy.

Data and Processes for Exploration

Chapter 5 reviewed evidence-based practice registries and the basis for rating the quality and extent of evidence, as well as for which populations an evidence-based practice may be appropriate. Chapter 6 reviewed a wide variety of evidence-based practices, as well as how a community might offer an integrated array of them. But how should such decisions be made?

A gaps analysis identifies the most substantial population concerns, as well as resources and services currently available. Population concerns can be identified from census data, arrests and incarceration data, data that identify neighborhoods with the highest number of child abuse and neglect reports, as well as school system academic reports, etc. It is important to examine these data through a variety of lenses. If only analyzed in aggregate, county or state data reports may not iden-

© Springer Nature Switzerland AG 2019   121
R. Bertram and S. Kerns, *Selecting and Implementing Evidence-Based Practice*,
https://doi.org/10.1007/978-3-030-11325-4_11

tify or may misrepresent concerns of specific neighborhoods with specific demographic and cultural composition, or they may fail to identify unique concerns of under-represented groups entirely. A 'data-informed' approach rather than a strict 'data-driven' approach allows for considerations of the local context and unique needs across diverse parts of the population. To illustrate this, Dr. Kerns will provide an example from one of her first experiences using data to inform evidence-based practice selection, using a model called Partnerships for Success (Julian, 2006).

Partnerships for Success: An Example

A number of years ago, I had the unique opportunity to leverage legislative funding to engage a community. This "community" was a tight-knit two-county geographic area interested in a process of selection and installation of evidence-based practices for children and adolescents. The entire story can be found in Kerns, Rivers and Enns (2009).

At the time this project started, the evidence-based practice movement was in its infancy. There were not yet well-established evidence-based practice registries to help guide identification of programs. Implementation science and frameworks were just beginning to emerge. I found myself with a dedicated group of individuals who had limited access to the peer-reviewed journals containing information about the effectiveness of specific practice or program models. As an academic, I had access to the journal articles, but needed to understand more about the community before I could help them carefully consider different models and offer suggestions for what might be appropriate to address their concerns. We used the Partnerships for Success model (Julian, 2006) to help guide the Pacific Northwest community in a thoughtful process of decision making. The main steps in Partnerships for Success are discussed below.

We first attended to community data sources. The exploration team included a core team of community members and academics. Community members represented the local behavioral healthcare organization responsible for Medicaid disbursement, a local community mental health agency and partner organization, and a representative from the court system. In addition to this core team, a broader stakeholder group convened as a resource to explore findings from a gaps analysis. It included family members, other community-based non-profit agencies, county commissioners, representatives of the faith-based community, Tribal leaders, child welfare professionals and others.

Project partner organizations used administrative data to identify how many children were currently being served by the community's system of services. They examined the types of diagnoses, the types of systems and number of organizations serving them, and the overall cost of service provision. Through this data-informed process, they were able to identify a subset of youth who were disproportionately costly within the system. These youth were multisystem involved and tended to be adolescents.

To better understand actual services that were currently available, we developed a survey that was administered to service agencies across the two-county area. An additional survey was developed for families to complete. This survey was made available in two community-based agencies; one agency was the only mental health agency that served the two-county area, and the other agency served youth and families with complex economic, educational, and behavioral health needs. Both surveys assessed the extent of available services.

With demographics, behaviors of concern and service availability information in hand, we identified community concerns and community-based resources. From this, we narrowed down the types of programs that would be most useful for these two counties, conducting a "gaps analysis" that articulated the community's unmet concerns (adolescent and youth substance use and antisocial behavior). We then strategically identified several different evidence-based programs that could potentially address this service gap. From that list of programs, we examined each against several criteria, including feasibility of implementation and alignment with the community's guiding principles. Ultimately, process resulted in the selection of Multisystemic Therapy as the evidence-based intervention that would best address this gap.

While this process resulted in identifying a program that clearly had the potential to meet community needs, if we had been entirely "data driven," we would have overlooked the Native American reservation needs. Because data across the two counties were aggregated and the population living on the reservation was very small compared to the rest of the community (~700 people), the unique needs of this population were masked within the overall data. Fortunately, we had a strong exploration team with representatives from that tribe who identified this oversight.

We slowed down and conducted a separate needs and resource analysis for the reservation community. Results demonstrated that priority needs were different for this community, namely substance abuse and trauma. The tribe already had a number of programs for addressing substance abuse, but lacked available treatments to address multigenerational trauma. The tribe ended up selecting Trauma-Focused Cognitive Behavioral Therapy (TF-CBT) as their evidence-based treatment of choice.

The exploration team explored whether the original TF-CBT would be appropriate or if a native adaptation of TF-CBT called Honoring Children Mending the Circle (BigFoot & Schmidt, 2010) would be better. Ultimately, the tribe decided to go with the original TF-CBT and to assess after a period of time if any accommodations were needed. The only adaptation identified was the manner in which the youth developed their trauma narrative. Because the tribe had a rich culture of creating canoe paddles and basket weaving as part of storytelling, they wanted to incorporate these forms of expression into the youth's trauma narrative. Treatment development experts were consulted, and it was determined that this accommodation should not impact the core components of TF-CBT. The youth were still completing trauma narratives. They were putting them into a cultural context that was meaningful. This project illustrates several important points about using data to inform program selection:

- Team composition should be carefully considered. Participants should include families and their natural supports, as well as service organizations.
- Community-specific data should be as broad and deep as possible. Information about community capabilities, values and strengths is as important as information about behaviors of concern.
- Disaggregating data (analyzing data separately by different demographic groups) can help identify needs of often overlooked sub-populations. Including representatives from those populations in the exploration process.
- Selection of evidence-based practices begins with identifying population needs and characteristics. Pairing that with resource assessment ensures that selection of evidence-based practices will address gaps in services.

Getting to Outcomes

Well-organized implementation planning processes provide accountability within an organization as well as between the organization, the community, and funding sources. Another model for organizing implementation is Abe Wandersman and colleagues Getting to Outcomes (Wandersman et al., 2000). Developed prior to the identification of the NIRN frameworks, this method helps communities and organizations achieve outcomes through a planful ten-step process that explores a number of questions (as listed in Wandersman et al., 2000):

- What are the underlying needs and resources that need to be addressed?
- What are the goals, target population, and objectives to address community needs and change the underlying conditions?
- Which science (evidence)-based models and best practice programs can be used to reach those goals?
- What actions need to be taken so that the selected program "Fits" the community context?
- What organizational capacities are needed to implement the intervention program?
- What is the plan for this program?
- How will the quality of implementation be assessed?
- How well did the program work?
- How will continuous quality improvement strategies be incorporated?
- If the program is successful, how will it be sustained?

As seen by this list of accountability questions, Getting to Outcomes overlays a thoughtful planning process with a meaningful evaluation process so that communities have a comprehensive system of supports enabling responsive feedback to funders and stakeholders.

Installing Implementation Feedback Loops

Once an organization selects a new practice model, its leadership and implementation team turn their attention to installation stage activities, aligning competency, and organizational drivers for high fidelity implementation and improved population outcomes. Leadership and the implementation team should install and monitor practice-informed-policy (PIP) and policy-enabled-practice (PEP) feedback loops.

As discussed in Chap. 8, model-pertinent criteria for staff selection, for training, and for the frequency, formats, and focus of coaching should be established. These adjustments should be integrated with organization policies and procedures. Leadership and the implementation team should identify what kinds of data can best inform how consistently these criteria are met. During implementation, by comparing these data with fidelity and eventually with client outcome data, organization leadership and the implementation team will be able to address challenges before they stall implementation. The use of technological resources for organizational improvement is increasingly expected and essential (Chorpita et al. 2008). When installation stage activities are fully addressed, an organization won't suffer costly "train and hope" discussed in Chap. 10.

Using Data to Guide Practice

The right data provide an incredibly useful means to assess client needs or behaviors of concern and to track client outcomes during the course of service delivery. With the growth of integrated care (e.g., Bickman, Lyon, & Wolpert, 2016; Bortranger & Lyon, 2015; Fortney et al., 2016) the use of symptom monitoring frameworks has gained momentum. These frameworks track symptoms over time. Clients complete a brief screening tool at the first session, and each session thereafter or on a pre-determined schedule. These behavioral data are entered into a data system that scores and tracks outcomes over time.

Practitioners use this information to determine if client symptoms are diminishing. These data also guide supervision and coaching. They can be used to identify emerging practitioner competence as well as to allow more time and focus to be placed on those clients who are not experiencing improvement. The data can be also be compared with fidelity data.

Symptom monitoring is a strategy that helps in development of individualized medicine (Ng & Weisz, 2016). Scott and Lewis (2015) provide a nice explanation of the potential of symptom monitoring as an enhancement for any evidence-based practice. Because most of these practices have an assessment strategy at the beginning of treatment, repeated measures of symptoms, and fidelity of practice provides highly useful feedback loops for coaching practitioner competence and confidence. These data, when combined with monitoring data on the consistency and quality of staff selection and training criteria, provide organization leadership and the implementation team with information needed to identify implementation challenges early to make adjustments.

Symptom monitoring can be low tech or higher tech. The lowest tech option is to have clients complete questionnaires during each session, hand score responses, and plot the scores on a graph. This has the advantage of being cost-effective but can take time out of a clinical session, especially if the measure is complex to score. There are relatively inexpensive websites that can help with symptom monitoring. One we use in several of our clinical implementation projects is the EBP toolkit (www.ebptoolkit.com). Agencies pay a one-time set-up fee (it is $500 as of 2018) and then just $.14 per user per day. PracticeWise (www.practicewise.com) is similar. In it, there is a wealth of resources including access to an Excel document that track symptoms and clinical activities over time. In 2018, the cost of this clinical dashboard was only $53. The main difference between these tools is that PracticeWise targets individual practitioner use while the EBP toolkit is designed to support supervision and consultation activities as well as symptoms and practice activities.

Another example of helpful data is the fidelity and outcomes dashboard used by teams delivering Multisystemic Therapy (MST). All licensed MST teams are required to use a website to enter clinical information about cases. These data are used to assess treatment fidelity and outcomes. Metrics such as caseload sizes, treatment duration, and fidelity scores inform how well teams are functioning as well as outcomes such as whether the youth is living at home at the end of treatment, whether they are in school or working, and if they have had any new arrests during the course of treatment. This helps MST teams to track what kinds of outcomes they are getting and if there are additional training needs. Tracking data in this way has an added advantage of enabling teams to share data with funding sources and agency partners to identify how the service site is functioning.

Summary

Well-organized implementation planning processes provide accountability within an organization as well as between the organization, the community, and funding sources. Well-composed implementation teams include leadership from key organizations with access to funding and resources, representatives from community-based agencies, as well as families, and other interested community representatives.

Establishing a common goal and objectives related to specific client populations helps organize pursuit of meaningful data to guide selection and placement of evidence-based programs. Established processes such as Getting to Outcomes, and the gaps analysis used in Partnerships for Success can provide guidelines for securing decision-making data.

Once a practice model is chosen, the implementation science and frameworks presented in Chaps. 8 and 9 identify specific activities, strategies, and processes for the installation and initial implementation of that evidence-based practice. Its effective implementation is not simply a matter of staff selection, training, and coaching. Those competency drivers of implementation should be monitored, informed, and guided by model-pertinent data feedback loops in which practice informs policy and policy can enable practice in continuous quality improvement in the fidelity and effectiveness of service delivery.

References

Bickman, L., Lyon, A. R., & Wolpert, M. (2016). Achieving precision mental health through effective assessment, monitoring, and feedback processes: Introduction to the special issue. *Administration and Policy in Mental Health and Mental Health Services Research, 43*(3), 271–276.

Bigfoot, D. S., & Schmidt, S. R. (2010). Honoring children, mending the circle: Cultural adaptation of trauma-focused cognitive-behavioral therapy for American Indian and Alaska Native children. *Journal of Clinical Psychology, 66*(8), 847–856.

Borntrager, C., & Lyon, A. R. (2015). Client progress monitoring and feedback in school-based mental health. *Cognitive and Behavioral Practice, 22*(1), 74–86.

Chorpita, B. F., Bernstein, A., Daleiden, E. L., & Research Network on Youth Mental Health. (2008). Driving with roadmaps and dashboards: Using information resources to structure the decision models in service organizations. *Administration and Policy in Mental Health and Mental Health Services Research, 35*(1–2), 114–123.

Fortney, J. C., Unützer, J., Wrenn, G., Pyne, J. M., Smith, G. R., Schoenbaum, M., et al. (2016). A tipping point for measurement-based care. *Psychiatric Services, 68*(2), 179–188.

Julian, D. A. (2006). A community practice model for community psychologists and some examples of the application of community practice skills from the partnerships for success initiative in Ohio. *American Journal of Community Psychology, 37*(1–2), 21–27.

Kerns, S. E. U., Rivers, A. M., & Enns, G. W. (2009). Partnerships for success in Washington State: Supporting evidence-based programming for children's mental health. *Report on Emotional and Behavioral Disorders in Youth, 9*, 55–62.

Ng, M. Y., & Weisz, J. R. (2016). Annual research review: Building a science of personalized intervention for youth mental health. *Journal of Child Psychology and Psychiatry, 57*(3), 216–236.

Scott, K., & Lewis, C. C. (2015). Using measurement-based care to enhance any treatment. *Cognitive and behavioral practice, 22*(1), 49–59.

Wandersman, A., Imm, P., Chinman, M., & Kaftarian, S. (2000). Getting to outcomes: A results-based approach to accountability. *Evaluation and Program Planning, 23*(3), 389–395.

Chapter 12
Pathways to the Future:
A Tale of Two Programs

> To introduce the integration of evidence-based practice and implementation science in academic courses and field curricula, this chapter begins with an allegorical tale of two programs in the community of Promiseville. We conclude with current examples of academic and behavioral healthcare program collaboration on pathways to a future shaped by science and exploration. Yes, even in these troubled times, some dare to go where few have gone before!

Once upon a time in the once pleasant community of Promiseville, middle and lower income families lost hope for the upward mobility of previous generations as a few well-to-do families become even more rich. Social and behavioral problems increased. Families fought. Gangs formed. Individual resident depression and anxiety rose.

The local behavioral healthcare (BHC) program provided services for the increasingly troubled residents of Promiseville. For the most part, BHC's clinicians functioned with relative autonomy using an eclectic range of techniques. Depending upon requirements of state and federal funding, BHC leadership focused upon different social or behavioral problems. When domestic violence gained legislative attention, they pursued grants describing how clinicians individualize service to address domestic violence victim needs. When antisocial youth behavior received legislative attention, BHC administrators pursued grants describing how clinicians individualize service based on youth and family needs and included a popular but untested parent training approach. With each new funding emphasis, BHC slightly adjusted or expanded its eclectic counseling approaches.

Promiseville's local university had a long-standing professional degree program (PDP). Its mission statement included statements about improving the lives of families in the urban community. Supporting this, its website touted the number of students that provided from 16 to 24 h a week of service to the community in their field learning sites. PDP students studied values and ethics, theories, and techniques. Upon graduation, they worked in a variety of settings, including the BHC clinic.

© Springer Nature Switzerland AG 2019
R. Bertram and S. Kerns, *Selecting and Implementing Evidence-Based Practice*,
https://doi.org/10.1007/978-3-030-11325-4_12

PDP faculty were a bit "long in the tooth." Many earned their degrees well before the economic stagnation and social problems were fully evident. The few faculty with more recent degrees tried to help their colleagues understand that as socioeconomic conditions deteriorated, practice shaped by science was emerging, developing evidence for specific treatment models, as well as how to best implement them.

Five years ago, in Promiseville, the words "synergistic" and "complementarity" would have been antonym descriptors of the relationship between PDP and BHC. Faculty in the academic program shaped curricula to address broadly described national accrediting requirements. Individual faculty were responsible for the content of each course, and once established, syllabi rarely changed. Field learning was not well-integrated with course content. The office of the field coordinator functioned like a silo in PDP's academic program. Field learning opportunities were broadly organized by types of setting. The coordinator believed that field sites were primarily interested in the unpaid service hours provided by a student. Field learning plans targeted the same broad competencies required of course curricula by the accrediting body. Individualizing and monitoring each student's learning activities in that plan were the responsibilities of a field liaison who did not teach academic courses. This occurred in one or two visits each semester with the student and the field instructor at the field site. There was little focus upon application of academic course content. Students reported their hours of field learning each month to the field office. The field liaison focused on competencies and activities in the learning plan and the field instructor–student relationship. When student or field instructor complaints or concerns arose, it strained the relationship between the field setting and the academic program's field office. Individual field instructors usually enjoyed developing students, but their managers and administrators sometimes wondered if it was worth lost time and occasional headaches.

The behavioral healthcare (BHC) program offered an array of individual, group, and family treatments for a variety of behaviors of concern. Much of its funding was sourced through the state's public child welfare system through long-standing federal legislation and funding. Over the years, BHC developed new services as other funding opportunities arose, usually from private foundations and occasionally from federal grants. As a result, the service array resembled a mosaic portrait from a decade of pursuing funding from different sources, each of which had a different focus and requirements. BHC was an approved field learning site for PDP with several field instructors, each responsible for a different type of service or service to a different population.

Thus, BHC and PDP functioned as mutually reinforcing yet relatively disengaged silos. BHC's mission statement was remarkably similar to PDP's assertions of service to Promiseville. Its website even identified the annual hours of treatment that BHC clinicians provided to the community's children, youth, and families. There were more than enough client concerns to keep BHC in business. There was more than enough need for new practitioners to maintain PDP enrollment. Although one or two PDP students might be placed for field learning experience in BHC's eclectic services, upon graduation they usually did not become BHC practitioners. Because BHC emphasized an individualized eclectic approach to client concerns, it never took the time to consider PDP's curriculum. And never the twain did meet (apologies to R. Kipling).

Recently, to align with federal funding guidelines, the state legislature required publicly funded service organizations to increasingly deliver evidence-based interventions. After five years, service organizations like BHC would have to ensure that at least 40% of clients received an evidence-based intervention matched to their clinical needs. This legislation allocated sufficient time and funds for a community planning process to identify the most appropriate evidence-based practices for specific needs and cultural contexts. Because insurance reimbursement increasingly rewarded use of evidence-based practice, BHC administrators had already been thinking of adding evidence-based treatments to upgrade their service array. This infusion of modest but helpful state funding was just what BHC needed for more targeted planning.

A new pathway in this tale of two programs then emerged. BHC convened a group of community stakeholders and a stratified sample of its staff early in this exploration and planning process. This group included representatives from the juvenile justice, education, child welfare, legal, philanthropic, and religious communities. Participants intentionally included prior clients who had successful treatment outcomes and successfully navigated the community's somewhat siloed system of services to reunite with their children or stay out of justice facilities. BHC also invited PDP's director to identify select faculty to participate in this stakeholder exploration and planning group. The director recognized this was an opportunity for the newer faculty with interests in evidence-based practice to discuss how they and select students might support and participate in these efforts.

Facilitated by BHC, the stakeholder group organized and conducted a comprehensive assessment that identified client diagnoses and the types of concerns most commonly reported, as well as community resources and types of services. Participating PDP faculty assigned graduate students to support analysis of the community assessment data. Using registries like Blueprints for Healthy Youth Development, the California Evidence-Based Clearinghouse for Child Welfare, the Cochrane Collaboration, and others, they cross-walked identified needs and concerns with possible evidence-based practices. The stakeholder group discussed the cultural relevance of these options and whether a practice might overlap with services provided in other settings. From this thorough community assessment, BHC identified three evidence-based practices for distinct behaviors of concern that would address the needs of approximately 65% of their current clients, thus enabling them to achieve the legislatively mandated goal. In close collaboration with current managers, supervisors, and practitioners, clinic leadership selected: (1) *Trauma-Focused Cognitive Behavior Therapy* for children and *Cognitive Processing Therapy* for adults—two related interventions focused on trauma; (2) *Parent–Child Interaction Therapy*—a parenting intervention that could be used for children referred to school and family behavior problems as well as for the mandated clients from the child welfare system who were required to participate in a parenting intervention; and (3) *Contingency Management*—a substance abuse-specific evidence-based practice that is appropriate for adolescents and adults.

BHC then initiated a comprehensive implementation planning process. Leadership and staff who participated in the exploration process comprised the organization's implementation team. Because the clinic had no experience with simultaneous implementation of so many new practices, it engaged an intermediary organization to ensure careful installation and systematic implementation of the three evidence-based practices. This included planful alignment of staff selection criteria and processes, developing initial training, identifying the frequency, formats, and focus of supervision, as well as how fidelity data would inform that coaching. They also reviewed and aligned internal agency policy and procedure. With support from the intermediary organization, BHC leadership organized its data system to monitor the percentage of clients receiving the three evidence-based services and the percentage that achieved improved outcomes.

As evidence-based practices become more prevalent, intermediary organizations emerged. They specialize in bringing knowledge and resources to address implementation needs with an organization. Technical assistance can address very practical concerns about case documentation or third-party reimbursement, as well as complex realignment of competency and organization drivers of implementation (Franks & Bory, 2015; Halle, Metz, & Martinez-Beck, 2013).

Because clinic staff engaged in the selection of the new practices, there was excitement about this new state-funded initiative. Though a few clinicians were skeptical, they were willing to try the new practices. Importantly, the clinic allowed practitioners to select which of the distinct evidence-based practices they wished to learn to provide. This helped tremendously with staff investment and interest in the new practice.

The intermediary organization helped the agency implementation team to carefully consider intake procedures and specify how clients would be identified for each new practice. The clinic created informational brochures about each of the new practices and translated them into the three most common languages spoken in the community. Intake staff were trained on how to engage clients about their choices in treatment as well as the clinical focus and expected outcomes for each new practice. Case documentation was modified to reinforce fidelity to the three evidence-based treatments. This documentation and the data system tracking client outcomes enabled supervisors to monitor and coach practitioner competence and treatment progress.

The staff in the implementation team worked with BHC leadership to determine performance-based incentives for the delivery of the evidence-based practices to the appropriate clients. Incentives increased with improvements in fidelity and outcomes. Prior to the initial training for each of the three practices, this implementation team worked collaboratively with the intermediary organization to define the training and consultation support plan with purveyors of each practice model. Together, they ensured that sufficient resources and time were allocated for managers, supervisors, and practitioners to participate in ongoing consultation and treatment fidelity supports.

In these installation stage discussions, they anticipated a major implementation challenge would be addressing workforce readiness to deliver these interventions after the initial training and support activities. This behavioral healthcare clinic experienced 20–30% staff turnover in any given year and would not have the subsequent resources to continually provide an intensive level of training.

Up until this point, the local academic program (PDP) had only participated in the local stakeholder meetings and enabled some graduate students to provide dedicated support during the needs assessment phase. However, now BHC leadership engaged PDP leadership with an invitation and a challenge: "Consistently provide us with a ready workforce." A new pathway to the future opened as together they closely examined PDP curriculum. While some courses presented content about a process of evidence-based practice as well as client trauma, no courses specifically prepared students to deliver the new practices identified by the clinic. Further, the faculty had limited knowledge or expertise in these specific practices and would likely be reluctant to teach specific practices without additional support.

The academic program's challenge was that their students could be placed at any number of local agencies, and once students graduate, they could take positions in other regions or even outside the state. How could PDP address this agency partner's need to better serve the community while also ensuring that students would graduate with knowledge and skill sets to work effectively in a variety of settings?

Working with BHC leadership, the PDP director engaged the field coordinator with the newer faculty that were versed in evidence-based practice and implementation science. Together, they planned and initiated a multiphased process to more fully integrate course content and assignments with field practicum experiences. As an initial step, they invited select faculty to join them in the clinic's initial training events. Participating faculty focused on mastering the core components of the practices, the populations for which they were most effective, and the practice model's theory of change.

Participating faculty realized that understanding key elements and activities of practice models, the populations best served by them, and their theory of change would be a beneficial framework for all practice courses so students would learn to think through these components to understand service delivery wherever they might be employed. Once mastered, PDP leadership engaged other faculties to ensure that courses on human behavior teach students the relationship between underlying theories and the common elements and activities in evidence-based practice. Research and policy course assignments were designed to ensure that students learned to search for and critically review the peer-reviewed literature as well as to search for proven practices in registries such as Blueprints for Healthy Youth Development and the California Evidence-Based Clearinghouse for Child Welfare.

In the BHC training events, participating faculty worked with the purveyors of each practice to identify specific classroom-based exercises that would engage students in learning critical elements and activities of each of the three evidence-based practices as well as skills in delivering them. Over time, some of these faculties developed a deeper interest in the evidence-based practice models and the university supported their participation in more advanced training for coaching and consultation. Two of these faculties eventually became accredited trainers, enabling them to blend the official training directly into their courses. These faculties also became a resource to BHC when it needed new staff training events or even booster training sessions for previously trained staff. This also provided additional income for these faculties as well as opportunities for applied research, presentations, and publishing opportunities about course development, training and consultation, and university—community collaboration.

As this initiative progressed, a streamlined process emerged for assigning students to BHC for targeted practicum experiences. Specifically, students were required to complete a fundamentals of evidence-based practice course in their first year of studies and then a course that presented specific evidence-based practices during the fall semester of their second year. For that semester, students could apply to be part of the state-funded BHC evidence-based practice initiative. If accepted, they were assigned a field practicum placement at the agency and given the opportunity to deliver evidence-based practices with clients. This essentially served as a clinical internship, and well-matched and performing students were offered postgraduate BHC employment. After one year of employment, BHC awarded them $1000 to help offset student loan expenses or to serve as a further incentive.

From the BHC's perspective, this was an efficient way to guarantee a well-selected and highly trained workforce. Over time, it could significantly reduce the costs of searching for, screening, selecting, and training new staff. From the academic program's perspective, they were able to upgrade faculty knowledge and skills with little additional cost. This made curricula more current with funding trends and community needs, and the selected students received a well-focused field practicum opportunity. Meanwhile, all PDP students were receiving more current knowledge and developing skills that made them more marketable upon graduation, and selected students had a field learning opportunity that could guarantee employment and a pathway to supervision hours required for licensure.

Promiseville now had an integrated approach for behavioral healthcare workforce development that targeted the specific needs of the community. Because of this symbiotic partnership's strong focus through implementation science to guide evidence-based practice installation and sustainability, both BHC and PDP programs grew over time and became well established. Even better, the community members of Promiseville now had access to high-quality evidence-based interventions for some of their most common areas of need. Substance abuse rates declined, fewer parents had their children removed due to abuse and neglect, and the school reported a decrease in behavioral concerns and disruptions.

This tale of two programs may sound idyllic, but in large and small ways it is occurring in some communities across the USA. Following the Barwick study (Barwick, 2011) and subsequent Child and Family Evidence-Based Practice Consortium study of MSW curricula (Bertram, Charnin, Kerns, & Long, 2015), a special issue of the Journal of Social Work Education was dedicated to exploring how to integrate evidence-based practice and implementation science into academic and field curricula (Bertram & Kerns, 2018). The call for abstracts yielded 55 proposed manuscripts, demonstrating a breadth of examples and interest in the field. Ultimately, 20 were invited for submission with ten exemplary articles finally reaching publication. Articles included examples from comprehensive curricular reform to smaller strategies of embedding specific evidence-based practices within a single course design, as well as how resources such as the California Evidence-Based Clearinghouse could provide comprehensive information about evidence-based practice for students and field agencies alike (Nwabuzor Ogbonnaya, Martin, & Walsh, 2018).

Here, we highlight two particularly vibrant examples. The first is an article by Mennen et al. (2018) in which they describe a comprehensive effort to leverage a large-scale community-based implementation to embed an intervention called Managing and Adapting Practice (MAP) into curricula. The MAP approach leverages PracticeWise (described in Chap. 11) to help guide practitioners to use evidence-based approaches that are determined a priori and that are based on the identification of clinical need. In this paper, the authors describe a comprehensive planning process that included a design team at the local university and a close partnership with the community-based agencies. At the community level, around 1700 practitioners in the local service area received training in MAP. At the university level, all of the course instructors were trained. Because they integrated this training into the core curriculum, nearly 250 students learned MAP and then practiced the intervention at their field placements!

Comprehensive integration of evidence-based practice and implementation science in both academic and field curricula at the University of Missouri–Kansas City School of Social Work was also part of this special issue (Bertram, Choi, & Elsen, 2018). The academic program had already transformed a required second-year MSW research course to teach students implementation science and frameworks by having them conduct an implementation evaluation of their field sites. Finding that there was all too often lack of clarity about practice models and consequent ineffective implementation led students to question the content of other courses. (Bertram, King, Pederson, & Nutt, 2014). New courses were developed that compared the development and implementation of Multisystemic Therapy with wraparound and other collaborative family-centered practices.

Finally, a National Child Welfare Workforce Initiative (NCWWI) University Partnership Grant provided the opportunity to transform field curricula using principles from implementation science. Selected students rotate through primary, secondary, and tertiary prevention services in public and private child welfare settings. Field learning plans focus through implementation science and frameworks. At the end of each week, a NCWWI cohort seminar integrates academic and field learning. Student's weekly field portfolios provide means to monitor learning and field instruction. Students are required to search for, critically analyze and share evidence-informed peer-reviewed literature related to each week's activities, and to share it with their field instructor. Three times a semester, field instructors meet to review the use of the literature at the site as well as field learning challenges and strategies. End of semester focus groups conducted separately with students and with field instructors identify what is working well and what requires adjustment. These structures and processes function as plan-do-study-act feedback loops for continuous improvement of instruction and student learning, while student products produced for the implementation evaluation course inform public and private child welfare organizations as they install and implement promising or evidence-based practices. Graduates are now performing as program specialists, trainers, and implementation managers in these organizations (Bertram et al., 2018; Bertram, Decker, Gillies, & Choi, 2017).

As seen in these two examples, when comprehensive efforts to select and implement evidence-based practices bridge academic programs and community services, the whole becomes greater than the sum of its parts. This is a promising and productive path to ensure that evidence-based practices are selected and implemented in a sustainable manner while simultaneously developing an evidence-based and implementation-informed workforce.

Future Pathways

The field of implementation science arose from the acknowledgment that much more is known about effective practice than is delivered in usual care settings. Implementation science guides sustainable adoption of effective practices. It supports the continued development of staff competence and confidence in the delivery of effective practices with fidelity. It supports sustainable, improved client outcomes.

However, a new gap is emerging. We now know more about effective implementation than what is used in practice settings. This must be addressed. It is incumbent upon those with knowledge of evidence-based practice and implementation science to identify how to make this knowledge quickly available in formats that are readily understood, practical, and usable. Development and investment in intermediary organizations can bridge this new gap between research and practice while leveraging the best of implementation science.

Logically, academic programs should play key roles in this process. However, as reported in Chap. 4 and spotlighted in this chapter's tale of two programs, some faculty of far too many academic programs are not sufficiently current in either evidence-based practice or implementation science. Where this is true, intermediary organizations and service organizations must actively engage academic programs and find ways to leverage more current and integrated academic and field curricula. The changing expectations of funding sources (see Chap. 3, discussion of Family First Prevention Services Act) will provide impetus. The integrated efforts of academic programs, intermediary organizations, and service organizations are ripe for faculty pursuit of grants for applied research, presentations, and publishing opportunities that are required academic responsibilities. Transformation of curricula can and must flow from such efforts.

There is a need for applied research examining contributing factors to the selection and implementation of evidence-based, research-based, or promising practices. Requirements of the Family First Prevention Services Act and related funding guidelines will provide many opportunities to study this. Implementation science has elucidated a number of critical factors necessary for effective practices to be embedded within organizations and their community contexts. However, the relative importance and the malleability of these factors have yet to be fully explored. For example, if the "host environment" (whether community or organization) appears inhospitable for evidence-based practice, what options are available and most effective to transform that environment?

Finally, implementation science and evidence-based practice continue to benefit from research that examines *what* works and *for whom*. *How do* psychosocial or behavioral interventions and especially implementation interventions work in diverse settings and with different populations? Empirical identification of the mechanisms of effectiveness (theory of change) will help to strategically tailor practice and implementation for different contexts and communities.

References

Barwick, M. (2011). Master's level clinician competencies in child and youth behavioral healthcare. *Emotional & Behavioral Disorders in Youth, 11*(2), 32–39.

Bertram, R. M., Charnin, L. A., Kerns, S. E. U., & Long, A. C. (2015). Evidence-based practices in North American MSW curricula. *Research on Social Work Practice, 25*(6), 737–748.

Bertram, R. M., Choi, S. W., & Elsen, M. (2018). Integrating implementation science and evidence-based practice into academic and field curricula. *Journal of Social Work Education*, 1–11.

Bertram, R. M., Decker, T., Gillies, M. E., & Choi, S. W. (2017). Transforming Missouri's child welfare system: Community conversations, organizational assessment, and university partnership. *Families in Society: The Journal of Contemporary Social Services, 98*(1), 9–17.

Bertram, R. & Kerns, S. E. U, guest editors (2018). Integrating evidence-based practice and implementation science into academic and field curricula. *Journal of Social Work Education, 54*(S1), 51–54.

Bertram, R. M., King, K., Pederson, R., & Nutt, J. (2014). Program implementation: An examination of the interface of curriculum and practice. *Journal of Evidence-Based Social Work, 11*, 193–207.

Franks, R. P., & Bory, C. T. (2015). Who supports the successful implementation and sustainability of evidence-based practices? Defining and understanding the roles of intermediary and purveyor organizations. *New Directions for Child and Adolescent Development, 149*, 41–56.

Halle, T., Metz, A., & Martinez-Beck, I. (Eds.). (2013). *Applying implementation science in early childhood programs and systems.* Paul H: Brookes Publishing Company.

Mennen, F. E., Cederbaum, J., Chorpita, B. F., Becker, K., Lopez, O., & Sela-Amit, M. (2018). The large-scale implementation of evidence-informed practice into a specialized MSW curriculum. *Journal of Social Work Education, 54*(S1), S56–S64.

Nwabuzor Ogbonnaya, I., Martin, J., & Walsh, C. R. (2018). Using the California evidence-based clearinghouse for child welfare as a tool for teaching evidence-based practice. *Journal of Social Work Education, 54*(sup1), S31–S40.

Appendix of Registries (Alphabetical)

Resource and website[a]	Advantages	Disadvantages
Blueprints for Healthy Youth Development http://www.blueprintsprograms.com/	Rigorous inclusion criteria; Searchable by population characteristics/needs Includes information on cost-benefit	Limited number of programs with smaller number of focus areas
California Evidence-Based Clearinghouse for Child Welfare http://www.cebc4cw.org/	Available information on a variety of topics related to evidence-based practices; Clear inclusion criteria; Provides scientific ratings to enable comparisons across programs; Contains ample information to facilitate early implementation planning	Programs evaluated predominately through a child welfare lens (may have limited broader applicability)
Crime Solutions https://www.crimesolutions.gov/	Searchable database with many search options; Able to sort based on evidence rating; Comprehensive glossary of terms	Programs evaluated predominately through a justice lens (may have limited broader applicability)
Home Visiting Evidence of Effectiveness (HomVEE) https://homvee.acf.hhs.gov/	Models are identified through a broad literature search Includes implementation profiles for all rated programs Requires a 1-year follow-up showing maintained treatment gains Can search by model, outcome domain, or rating	Somewhat less rigorous requirements for being deemed evidence-based; Programs focus on home visiting interventions for pregnant women and children birth through age 5 only (may have limited broader applicability)

(continued)

© Springer Nature Switzerland AG 2019
R. Bertram and S. Kerns, *Selecting and Implementing Evidence-Based Practice*,
https://doi.org/10.1007/978-3-030-11325-4

(continued)

Resource and website[a]	Advantages	Disadvantages
OJJDP Model Programs Guide https://www.ojjdp.gov/mpg/	Similar database look and feel as crime solutions (both justice-focused; use same database for youth programs); Inclusive of prevention and intervention programs	Programs evaluated predominately through a justice lens (may have limited broader applicability)
PracticeWise common components https://www.practicewise.com/	One-stop shop for information related to common elements of EBPs; Clinician tools; Web-based dashboard to track clinical progress	Subscription fee
SAMHSA's National Registry of Evidence-Based Programs and Practices http://www.nrepp.samhsa.gov/ Closed in January 2017 See: Green-Hennessy, 2018	Prior to closure provided comprehensive list of interventions; Many research references; Standardized ratings across multiple programs	Programs did not always meet evidence-based or research-based criteria discussed in Chap. 3
Washington State Institute for Public Policy (adult) https://www.wsipp.wa.gov/ReportFile/1644/Wsipp_Updated-Inventory-of-Evidence-based-Research-based-and-Promising-Practices-Prevention-and-Intervention-Services-for-Adult-Behavioral-Health_Report.pdf (child/youth) https://www.wsipp.wa.gov/ReportFile/1639/Wsipp_Updated-Inventory-of-Evidence-Based-Researched-Based-and-Promising-Practices-For-Prevention-and-Intervention-Services-for-Children-and-Juveniles-in-the-Child-Welfare-Juvenile-Justice-and-Mental-Health-Systems_Report.pdf	Clear definitions; Cost-benefit information available; Programs categorized by domain (e.g., juvenile justice, mental health, substance abuse)	Not easily searchable (lists are in PDF format, not an interactive Web site)

[a]Note, these websites (except NREPP) were active as of the end of 2018, but are subject to change. Some registries, like NREPP, lose funding and therefore are no longer available. New registries, such as the one being developed to support the Family First Prevention Services Act (FFPSA), are not yet available, but likely will be by the time this book is published

Complete References

Aarons, G. A., Green, A. E., Trott, E., Willging, C. E., Torres, E. M., Ehrhart, M. G., et al. (2016). The roles of system and organizational leadership in system-wide evidence-based intervention sustainment: A mixed-method study. *Administration and Policy in Mental Health and Mental Health Services Research, 43*(6), 991–1008.

Aarons, G. A., Hurlburt, M., & Horwitz, S. M. (2011). Advancing a conceptual model of evidence-based practice implementation in public service sectors. *Administration and Policy in Mental Health and Mental Health Services Research, 38*(1), 4–23.

Aarons, G. A., Sommerfeld, D., Hecht, D., Silovsky, J., & Chaffin, M. (2009). The impact of evidence-based practice implementation and fidelity monitoring on staff turnover: Evidence for a protective effect. *Journal of Consulting & Clinical Psychology, 77*(2), 270–280.

Aarons, G. A., & Sawitzky, A. C. (2006). Organizational culture and climate and mental health provider attitudes toward evidence-based practice. *Psychological Services, 3*(1), 61.

Addis, M., Wade, W. A., & Hatgis, C. (1999). Barriers to dissemination of evidence-based practices: Addressing practitioners' concerns about manual-based psychotherapies. *Clinical Psychology: Science and Practice, 6*, 430–441.

Alexander, J., Barton, C., Gordon, D., Grotpeter, J., Hansson, K., Harrison, R., et al. (1998). *Blueprints for violence prevention, book three: Functional family therapy.* Boulder, CO: Center for the Study and Prevention of Violence.

American Association for Marriage and Family Therapists. (2004). *Marriage and family therapy core competencies.* Retrieved from www.aamft.org.

American Psychological Association Presidential Task Force on Evidence Based-Practice. (2006). Evidence-based practice in psychology. *American Psychologist, 61*(4), 271-285. https://doi.org/10.1037/0003-066x.61.4.271.

Ardito, R. B., & Rabellino, D. (2011). Therapeutic alliance and outcome of psychotherapy: Historical excursus, measurements, and prospects for research. *Frontiers in Psychology, 2*, 270.

Balas, E. A., & Boren, S. A. (2000). Managing clinical knowledge for health care improvement. *Yearbook of Medical Informatics 2000: Patient-Centered Systems, (1).* 65-70.

Barth, R. P., Lee, B. R., Lindsey, M. A., Collins, K. S., Strieder, F., Chorpita, B. F., et al. (2012). Evidence-based practice at a crossroads: The timely emergence of common elements and common factors. *Research on Social Work Practice, 22*(1), 108–119.

Barwick, M. (2011). Master's level clinician competencies in child and youth behavioral healthcare. *Emotional & Behavioral Disorders in Youth, 11*(2), 32-29.

Beidas, R. S., Barmish, A. J., & Kendall, P. C. (2009). Training as usual: Can therapist behavior change after reading a manual and attending a brief workshop on cognitive behavioral therapy for youth anxiety? *Behavior Therapist, 32*(5), 97–101.

© Springer Nature Switzerland AG 2019
R. Bertram and S. Kerns, *Selecting and Implementing Evidence-Based Practice,*
https://doi.org/10.1007/978-3-030-11325-4

Bernal, G., Jiménez-Chafey, M. I., & Domenech Rodríguez, M. M. (2009). Cultural adaptation of treatments: A resource for considering culture in evidence-based practice. *Professional Psychology: Research and Practice, 40*(4), 361.

Bernet, A. C., Willens, D. E., & Bauer, M. S. (2012). Effectiveness-implementation hybrid designs: implications for quality improvement science. *Implementation Science, 8*(Suppl 1), S2.

Bertram, R. M., Blase, K. A., & Fixsen, D. L. (2015). Improving programs and outcomes: Implementation frameworks and organization change. *Research on Social Work Practice, 25* (4), 477–487.

Bertram, R., Blase, K., Shern, D., Shea, P., & Fixsen, D. (2011). *Policy research brief: Implementation opportunities and challenges for prevention and promotion initiatives.* Alexandria, VA: National Association of State Mental Health Program Directors (NASMHPD).

Bertram, R. M., Charnin, L. A., Kerns, S. E. U., & Long, A. C. (2015). Evidence-based practices in North American MSW curricula. *Research on Social Work Practice, 25*(6), 737–748.

Bertram, R. M., Choi, S. W., & Elsen, M. (2018). Integrating implementation science and evidence-based practice into academic and field curricula. *Journal of Social Work Education,* 1-11.

Bertram, R. M., Decker, T., Gillies, M. E., & Choi, S. W. (2017). Transforming Missouri's child welfare system: Community conversations, organizational assessment, and university partnership. *Families in Society: The Journal of Contemporary Social Services, 98*(1), 9–17.

Bertram, R. & Kerns, S. E. U, guest editors (2018). Integrating evidence-based practice and implementation science into academic and field curricula. *Journal of Social Work Education, 54*(S1), 51-54.

Bertram, R. M., King, K., Pederson, R., & Nutt, J. (2014). Program implementation: An examination of the interface of curriculum and practice. *Journal of Evidence-Based Social Work, 11,* 193–207.

Bertram, R. M., Schaffer, P., & Charnin, L. (2014). Changing organization culture: Data driven participatory evaluation and revision of wraparound implementation. *Journal of Evidence-Based Social Work, 11,* 18–29.

Bettinger, E. P., & Long, B. T. (2010). Does cheaper mean better? The impact of using adjunct instructors on student outcomes. *The Review of Economics and Statistics, 92*(3), 598–613.

Bickman, L., Lyon, A. R., & Wolpert, M. (2016). Achieving precision mental health through effective assessment, monitoring, and feedback processes: Introduction to the special issue. *Administration and Policy in Mental Health and Mental Health Services Research, 43*(3), 271–276.

Bigfoot, D. S., & Schmidt, S. R. (2010). Honoring children, mending the circle: cultural adaptation of trauma-focused cognitive-behavioral therapy for American Indian and Alaska Native children. *Journal of Clinical Psychology, 66*(8), 847–856.

BigFoot, D. S., & Funderburk, B. W. (2011). Honoring children, making relatives: The cultural translation of parent-child interaction therapy for American Indian and Alaska Native families. *Journal of Psychoactive Drugs, 43*(4), 309–318.

Blase, K. A., Van Dyke, M., Fixsen, D. L., & Wallace Bailey, F. (2012). Implementation science: Key concepts, themes, and evidence for practitioners in educational psychology. In B. Kelly & D. Perkins (Eds.), *Handbook of implementation science for psychology in education* (pp. 13–34). London: Cambridge University Press.

Borntrager, C., & Lyon, A. R. (2015). Client progress monitoring and feedback in school-based mental health. *Cognitive and Behavioral Practice, 22*(1), 74–86.

Bowen, M. (1978). *Family Therapy in Clinical Practice.* NY and London: Jason Aronson.

Bruns, E. J. (2008). The evidence base and wraparound. In E. J. Bruns & J. S. Walker (Eds.), *The resource guide to wraparound.* Portland, OR: National Wraparound Initiative, Research and Training Center for Family Support and Children's Mental Health.

Bruns, E. J., Kerns, S. E. U., Pullmann, M. D., Hensley, S. W., Lutterman, T., & Hoagwood, K. E. (2015). Research, data, and evidence-based treatment use in state behavioral health systems, 2001–2012. *Psychiatric Services, 67*(5), 496–503.

Bruns, E. J., Pullmann, M. D., Sather, A., Brinson, R. D., & Ramey, M. (2015). Effectiveness of wraparound versus case management for children and adolescents: Results of a randomized study. *Administration and Policy in Mental Health and Mental Health Services Research, 42* (3), 309–322.

Carroll, C., Patterson, M., Wood, S., Booth, A., Rick, J., & Balain, S. (2007). A conceptual framework for implementation fidelity. *Implementation science, 2*(1), 40.

Castro, F. G., Barrera, M., Jr., & Holleran Steiker, L. K. (2010). Issues and challenges in the design of culturally adapted evidence-based interventions. *Annual Review of Clinical Psychology, 6,* 213–239.

Chambless, D. L., & Hollon, S. D. (1998). Defining empirically supported therapies. *Journal of Consulting and Clinical Psychology, 66,* 7–18.

Chambless, D. L., & Ollendick, T. H. (2001). Empirically supported psychological interventions: Controversies and evidence. *Annual Review of Psychology, 52,* 685–716.

Chorpita, B. F., Bernstein, A., Daleiden, E. L., & Research Network on Youth Mental Health. (2008). Driving with roadmaps and dashboards: Using information resources to structure the decision models in service organizations. *Administration and Policy in Mental Health and Mental Health Services Research, 35*(1–2), 114–123.

Chorpita, B. F., Daleiden, E., & Weisz, J. R. (2005). Identifying and selecting the common elements of evidence based interventions: A distillation and matching model. *Mental Health Services Research, 7,* 5–20.

Chorpita, B. F., Becker, K. D., & Daleiden, E. L. (2007). Understanding the common elements of evidence based practice: Misconceptions and clinical examples. *Journal of the American Academy of Child and Adolescent Psychiatry, 46,* 647–652.

Chu, J., Leino, A., Pflum, S., & Sue, S. (2016). A model for the theoretical basis of cultural competency to guide psychotherapy. *Professional Psychology: Research and Practice, 47*(1), 18.

Cohen, J. A., Mannarino, A. P., & Deblinger, E. (2016). *Treating trauma and traumatic grief in children and adolescents.* Guilford Publications.

Commission on Accreditation for Marriage and Family Therapy Education. (2017). *Accreditation standards: Graduate & post-graduate marriage and family therapy training programs,* version 12.0. Alexandria, VA: Author.

Cook, J. R., Hausman, E. M., Jensen-Doss, A., & Hawley, K. M. (2017). Assessment practices of child clinicians: Results from a national survey. *Assessment, 24*(2), 210–221.

Council on Social Work Education. (2015). *Educational policy and accreditation standards.* Alexandria, VA: Author.

Crane, D. R., Wampler, K. S., Sprenkle, D. H., Sandberg, J. G., & Hovestadt, A. J. (2002). The scientist-practitioner model in marriage and family therapy doctoral programs. *Journal of Marital and Family Therapy, 28,* 75–83.

Crane, R. S., Kuyken, W., Williams, J. M. G., Hastings, R. P., Cooper, L., & Fennell, M. J. (2012). Competence in teaching mindfulness-based courses: concepts, development and assessment. *Mindfulness, 3*(1), 76–84.

Daly, A. J., & Chrispeels, J. (2008). A question of trust: Predictive conditions for adaptive and technical leadership in educational contexts. *Leadership and Policy in Schools, 7*(1), 30–63.

Damschroder, L. J., Aron, D. C., Keith, R. E., Kirsh, S. R., Alexander, J. A., & Lowery, J. C. (2009). Fostering implementation of health services research findings into practice: A consolidated framework for advancing implementation science. *Implementation science, 4*(1), 50.

Dopp, A. R., Borduin, C. M., Wagner, D. V., & Sawyer, A. M. (2014). The economic impact of multisystemic therapy through midlife: A cost–benefit analysis with serious juvenile offenders and their siblings. *Journal of Consulting and Clinical psychology, 82*(4), 694.

Dopp, A. R., Coen, A. S., Smith, A. B., Reno, J., Bernstein, D. H., Kerns, S. E. U., et al. (2018). Economic impact of the statewide implementation of an evidence-based treatment: Multisystemic therapy in New Mexico. *Behavior Therapy, 49*(4), 551–566.

Dorsey, S., Berliner, L., Lyon, A. R., Pullmann, M. D., & Murray, L. K. (2016). A statewide common elements initiative for children's mental health. *The Journal of Behavioral Health Services & Research, 43*(2), 246–261.

Dorsey, S., McLaughlin, K. A., Kerns, S. E. U., Harrison, J. P., Lambert, H. K., Briggs-King, E., et al. (2017). Evidence base update for psychosocial treatments for children and adolescents exposed to traumatic events. *Journal of Clinical Child and Adolescent Psychology, 46*(3), 303–330. https://doi.org/10.1080/15374416.2016.1220309.

Dorsey, S., Pullmann, M. D., Deblinger, E., Berliner, L., Kerns, S. E., Thompson, K., ... & Garland, A. F. (2013). Improving practice in community-based settings: A randomized trial of supervision–study protocol. *Implementation Science, 8*(1), 89.

Dorsey, S., Pullmann, M. D., Kerns, S. E., Jungbluth, N., Meza, R., Thompson, K., et al. (2017). The juggling act of supervision in community mental health: Implications for supporting evidence-based treatment. *Administration and Policy in Mental Health and Mental Health Services Research, 44*(6), 838–852.

Drabick, D. A., & Goldfried, M. R. (2000). Training the scientist– practitioner for the 21st century: Putting the bloom back on the rose. *Journal of Clinical Psychology, 56,* 327–340.

Duncan, B. L., Miller, S. D., Wampold, B. E., & Hubble, M. A. (2010). *The heart and soul of change: Delivering what works* (2nd ed.). Washington, DC: American Psychological Association.

Eaton, D. (2015). Making the shift: Leading first with who we are, not what we do. *People and Strategy, 38*(3), 46.

Epstein, M. H., Kutash, K. E., & Duchnowski, A. E. (1998). *Outcomes for children and youth with emotional and behavioral disorders and their families: Programs and evaluation best practices*. Pro-Ed.

Eyberg, S. M., Funderburk, B. W., Hembree-Kigin, T. L., McNeil, C. B., Querido, J. G., & Hood, K. K. (2001). Parent-child interaction therapy with behavior problem children: One and two year maintenance of treatment effects in the family. *Child & Family Behavior Therapy, 23*(4), 1–20.

Fixsen, D. L., Blase, K. A., Naoom, S. F., & Wallace, F. (2009). Core implementation components. *Research on Social Work Practice, 19*(5), 531–540.

Fixsen, D. L., Naoom, S. F., Blase, K. A., Friedman, R. M., & Wallace, F. (2005). *Implementation research: A synthesis of the literature*. Tampa, FL: University of South Florida, Louis de la Parte Florida Mental Health Institute, The National Implementation Research Network (FMHI Publication #231).

Frank, G. (1984). The Boulder Model: History, rationale, and critique. *Professional Psychology: Research and Practice, 15,* 417–435.

Franks, R. P., & Bory, C. T. (2015). Who supports the successful implementation and sustainability of evidence-based practices? Defining and understanding the roles of intermediary and purveyor organizations. *New Directions for Child and Adolescent Development, 149,* 41–56.

Franks, R. P., & Bory, C. T. (2017). Strategies for developing intermediary organizations: Considerations for practice. *Families in Society: The Journal of Contemporary Social Services, 98*(1), 27–34.

Foa, E. B., Hembree, E. A., Cahill, S. P., Rauch, S. A., Riggs, D. S., Feeny, N. C., et al. (2005). Randomized trial of prolonged exposure for posttraumatic stress disorder with and without cognitive restructuring: Outcome at academic and community clinics. *Journal of Consulting and Clinical psychology, 73*(5), 953.

Foa, E. B., Keane, T. M., Friedman, M. J., & Cohen, J. A. (Eds.). (2008). *Effective treatments for PTSD: Practice guidelines from the international society for traumatic stress studies.* Guilford Press.

Forehand, R., Dorsey, S., Jones, D. J., Long, N., & McMahon, R. J. (2010). Adherence and flexibility: They can (and do) coexist! *Clinical Psychology: Science and Practice, 17*(3), 258–264.

Fortney, J. C., Unützer, J., Wrenn, G., Pyne, J. M., Smith, G. R., Schoenbaum, M., et al. (2016). A tipping point for measurement-based care. *Psychiatric Services, 68*(2), 179–188.

Funderburk, B. W., & Eyberg, S. (2011). Parent–child interaction therapy. In J. C. Norcross, G. R. VandenBos, & D. K. Freedheim (Eds.), *History of psychotherapy: Continuity and change* (pp. 415–420). Washington, DC, US: American Psychological Association.

Gambrill, E. (1999). Evidence-based practice: An alternative to authority-based practice. *Families in Society: The Journal of Contemporary Human Services, 80,* 341–350. https://doi.org/10.1606/1044-3894.1214.

Gambrill, E. (2007). Views of evidence-based practice: Social workers' code of ethics and accreditation standards as guides for choice. *Journal of Social Work Education, 43,* 447–462.

Gambrill, E., & Gibbs, L. (2009). Developing well-structured questions for evidence-informed practice. In A. R. Roberts (Ed.), *Social workers' desk reference* (2nd ed., pp. 1120–1126). New York, NY: Oxford University Press.

Gambrill, E. (2010). Evidence-informed practice: Antidote to propaganda in the helping profession. *Research on Social Work Practice, 20,* 302–320.

Gambrill, E. (2018). Contributions of the process of evidence-based practice to implementation: Educational opportunities. *Journal of Social Work Education, 54*(sup1), S113–S125.

Gibbs, L., & Gambrill, E. (2002). Evidence-based practice: Counterarguments to objections. *Research on Social Work Practice, 12*(3), 452–476.

George, P., Kanary, P. J., Wotring, J., Bernstein, D., & Carter, W. J. (2008). *Financing evidence-based programs and practices: Changing systems to support effective service.* Denver, CO: Child and Family Evidence-Based Practice Consortium.

Gitterman, A., & Knight, C. (2013). Evidence-guided practice: Integrating the science and art of social work. *Families in Society: The Journal of Contemporary Social Services, 94,* 70–78.

Green, L. W. (2008). Making research relevant: If it is an evidence-based practice, where's the practice-based evidence?. *Family Practice, 25*(suppl_1), i20-i24.

Green-Hennessy, S. (2018). Suspension of the national registry of evidence-based programs and practices: The importance of adhering to the evidence. *Substance Abuse Treatment, Prevention, and Policy, 13*(1), 26.

Gregersen, E. (2009). *An Explorer's Guide to the Universe.* Rosen Publishing Group.

Haley, J. (1987). *The Jossey-Bass social and behavioral science series. Problem-solving therapy* (2nd ed.). San Francisco, CA, US: Jossey-Bass.

Halle, T., Metz, A., & Martinez-Beck, I. (Eds.). (2013). *Applying implementation science in early childhood programs and systems.* Paul H: Brookes Publishing Company.

Hawkins, J. D., Catalano, R. F., & Kuklinski, M. R. (2014). Communities that care. In *Encyclopedia of criminology and criminal justice.* (pp. 393-408). Springer, New York, NY.

Heifetz, R. A., & Laurie, D. L. (1997). The work of leadership. *Harvard business review, 75,* 124–134.

Henggeler, S. W., Schoenwald, S. K., Borduin, C. M., Rowland, M. D., & Cunningham, P. B. (2009). *Multisystemic Therapy for Anti-Social Behavior in Children and Adolescents* (2nd ed.). New York: Guilford Press.

Henggeler, S. W., Rowland, M. D., Randall, J., Ward, D. M., Pickrel, S. G., Cunningham, P. B., … & Santos, A. B. (1999). Home-based multisystemic therapy as an alternative to the hospitalization of youths in psychiatric crisis: Clinical outcomes. *Journal of the American Academy of Child & Adolescent Psychiatry, 38*(11), 1331-1339.

Hoge, M. A., Morris, J. A., Daniels, A. S., Huey, L. Y., Stuart, G. W., Adams, N., … & Storti, S. A. (2005). Report of recommendations: The Annapolis coalition conference on behavioral health work force competencies. *Administration and Policy in Mental Health and Mental Health Services Research, 32*(5-6), 651-663.

Hogue, A., Henderson, C. E., Dauber, S., Barajas, P. C., Fried, A., & Liddle, H. A. (2008). Treatment adherence, competence, and outcome in individual and family therapy for adolescent behavior problems. *Journal of Consulting and Clinical Psychology, 76*(4), 544–555.

Howard, M. O., McMillen, J. C., & Pollio, D. E. (2003). Teaching evidence-based practice: Toward a new paradigm for social work education. *Journal of Research on Social Work Practice, 13,* 234–259.

Hudson, C. (2009). Decision-making in evidence-based practice: Science and art. *Smith College Studies in Social Work, 79*, 155–174.

Huey, S. J., Jr., & Polo, A. J. (2008). Evidence-based psychosocial treatments for ethnic minority youth. *Journal of Clinical Child & Adolescent Psychology, 37*(1), 262–301.

Insel, T. (2015, July 14). Post by former NIMH director Thomas Insel: Quality counts [Blog post]. Retrieved from https://www.nimh.nih.gov/about/directors/thomas- insel/blog/2015/quality-counts. shtml.

Institute of Medicine. (2001). *Crossing the quality chasm: A new healthy system for the 21st Century*. Washington, DC: National Academic Press.

Institute of Medicine. (2015). *Psychosocial interventions for mental and substance use disorders: A framework for establishing evidence-based standards*. Washington, DC: The National Academies Press.

Julian, D. A. (2006). A community practice model for community psychologists and some examples of the application of community practice skills from the partnerships for success initiative in Ohio. *American Journal of Community Psychology, 37*(1–2), 21–27.

Kaminski, J. W., Valle, L. A., Filene, J. H., & Boyle, C. L. (2008). A meta-analytic review of components associated with parent training program effectiveness. *Journal of Abnormal Child Psychology, 36*(4), 567–589.

Kanary, P. J., Bertram, R. M., & Bernstein, D. (2017). The child and family evidence-based practice consortium: Pathways to the future. *Families in Society: The Journal of Contemporary Social Services, 98*(1), 7–8.

Karam, E. A., & Sprenkle, D. H. (2010). The research-informed clinician: A guide to training the next generation MFT. *Journal of Marital and Family Therapy, 36*(3), 307–319.

Kaslow, N. J., Rubin, N. J., Forrest, L., Elman, N. S., Van Horne, B. A., Jacobs, S. C., et al. (2007). Recognizing, assessing, and intervening with problems of professional competence. *Professional Psychology: Research and Practice, 38*(5), 479–492.

Kazdin, A. E., Bass, D., Ayers, W. A., & Rodgers, A. (1990). Empirical and clinical focus of child and adolescent psychotherapy research. *Journal of Consulting and Clinical Psychology, 58*(6), 729–740.

Kendall, P. C. (2006). *Coping cat workbook*. (2nd ed.). Workbook Publishing.

Kendall, P. C., Crawford, E. A., Kagan, E. R., Furr, J. M., & Podell, J. L. (2003). Child-focused treatment of anxiety. In J.R. Weisz, & A. E. Kazdin, (Eds.), *Evidence-Based Psychotherapies for Children and Adolescents*. (3rd ed., pp 81-100). Guilford Press.

Kerns, S. E. U., Bertram, R., Cannata, E., Marlowe, D. B., Wolfe, S. & Choi, S. W. (in progress). Evidence-based practice in masters of marriage and family therapy degree programs.

Kerns, S. E. U., Levin, C., Leith, J., Carey, C., & Uomoto, A. (2016). *Preliminary estimate of costs associated with implementing research and evidence-based practices for children and youth in Washington State (Report)*. University of Washington School of Medicine, Division of Public Behavioral Health and Justice Policy. Retrieved from https://www.hca.wa.gov/assets/program/ ebt-cost-study-report.pdf.

Kerns, S. E. U., McCormick, E., Negrete, A., Carey, C., Haaland, W., & Waller, S. (2017). Predicting post-training implementation of a parenting intervention. *Journal of Children's Services, 12*(4), 302–315.

Kerns, S. E. U., Rivers, A. M., & Enns, G. W. (2009). Partnerships for success in Washington State: Supporting evidence-based programming for children's mental health. *Report on Emotional and Behavioral Disorders in Youth, 9*, 55–62.

Kirk, M. A., Kelley, C., Yankey, N., Birken, S. A., Abadie, B., & Damschroder, L. (2015). A systematic review of the use of the consolidated framework for implementation research. *Implementation Science, 11*(1), 72.

Kutash, K., & Rivera, V. R. (1996). *What works in children's mental health services?: Uncovering answers to critical questions* (Vol. 3). Paul H Brookes Publishing Company.

Lau, A. S. (2006). Making the case for selective and directed cultural adaptations of evidence-based treatments: Examples from parent training. *Clinical Psychology: Science and Practice, 13*(4), 295–310.

Letourneau, E. J., Henggeler, S. W., Borduin, C. M., Schewe, P. A., McCart, M. R., Chapman, J. E., et al. (2009). Multisystemic therapy for juvenile sexual offenders: 1-year results from a randomized effectiveness trial. *Journal of Family Psychology, 23*, 89–102.

Lieberman, A. F., Van Horn, P., & Ippen, C. G. (2005). Toward evidence-based treatment: Child-parent psychotherapy with preschoolers exposed to marital violence. *Journal of the American Academy of Child & Adolescent Psychiatry, 44*(12), 1241–1248.

Lipsey, M. W. (2009). The primary factors that characterize effective interventions with juvenile offenders: A meta-analytic overview. *Victims and offenders, 4*(2), 124–147.

Lucock, M., Leach, C., Iveson, S., Lynch, K., Horsefield, C., & Hall, P. (2003). A systematic approach to practice-based evidence in a psychological therapies service. *Clinical Psychology & Psychotherapy: An International Journal of Theory & Practice, 10*(6), 389–399.

Lyon, A. R., Stirman, S. W., Kerns, S. E. U., & Bruns, E. J. (2011). Developing the mental health workforce: Review and application of training approaches from multiple disciplines. *Administration and Policy in Mental Health and Mental Health Services Research, 38*(4), 238–253.

Mazzucchelli, T. G., & Sanders, M. R. (2010). Facilitating practitioner flexibility within an empirically supported intervention: Lessons from a system of parenting support. *Clinical Psychology: Science and Practice, 17*(3), 238–252.

McMahon, R. J., & Forehand, R. L. (2005). *Helping the noncompliant child: Family-based treatment for oppositional behavior*. Guilford Press.

Mennen, F. E., Cederbaum, J., Chorpita, B. F., Becker, K., Lopez, O., & Sela-Amit, M. (2018). The large-scale implementation of evidence-informed practice into a specialized MSW curriculum. *Journal of Social Work Education, 54*(S1), S56–S64.

Metz, A., & Bartley, L. (2012). Active implementation frameworks for program success: How to use implementation science to improve outcomes for children. *Zero to Three Journal, 34*(4), 11–18.

Meyer, A. S., Templeton, G. B., Stinson, M. A., & Codone, S. (2016). Teaching research methods to MFT master's students: A comparison between scientist-practitioner and research-informed approaches. *Contemporary Family Therapy, 38*(3), 295–306.

Miller, W. R., & Rollnick, S. (2012). *Motivational interviewing: Helping people change*. Guilford press.

Minuchin, S. (1974). *Families & Family Therapy*. Cambridge, MA: Harvard University Press.

Minuchin, S., Montalvo, B., Guerney, B., Rosman, B., & Schumer, F. (1967). *Families of the slums*. New York: Basic Books.

Minuchin, S., & Fishman, H. C. (1981). *Family therapy techniques*. Cambridge, MA: Harvard University Press.

Morawska, A., Sanders, M., Goadby, E., Headley, C., Hodge, L., McAuliffe, C., ... & Anderson, E. (2011). Is the Triple P-Positive Parenting Program acceptable to parents from culturally diverse backgrounds?. *Journal of Child and Family Studies, 20*(5), 614-622.

Morawska, A., Sanders, M. R., O'Brien, J., McAuliffe, C., Pope, S., & Anderson, E. (2012). Practitioner perceptions of the use of the Triple P-Positive Parenting Program with families from culturally diverse backgrounds. *Australian Journal of Primary Health, 18*(4), 313–320.

Mufson, L., & Moreau, D. (1999). Interpersonal psychotherapy for depressed adolescents (IPT-A). *Handbook of psychotherapies with children and families* (pp. 239–253). Boston, MA: Springer.

Nelson, T. S., Chenail, R. J., Alexander, J. F., Crane, D. R., Johnson, S. M., & Schwallie, L. (2007). The development of core competencies for the practice of marriage and family therapy. *Journal of Marital and Family Therapy, 33*(4), 417–438.

Ng, M. Y., & Weisz, J. R. (2016). Annual Research Review: Building a science of personalized intervention for youth mental health. *Journal of Child Psychology and Psychiatry, 57*(3), 216–236.

Nilsen, P. (2015). Making sense of implementation theories, models and frameworks. *Implementation Science, 10*(1), 53.

Novins, D. K., Green, A. E., Legha, R. K., & Aarons, G. A. (2013). Dissemination and implementation of evidence-based practices for child and adolescent mental health: A systematic review. *Journal of the American Academy of Child & Adolescent Psychiatry, 52* (10), 1009–1025.

Nowak, C., & Heinrichs, N. (2008). A comprehensive meta-analysis of Triple P-Positive Parenting Program using hierarchical linear modeling: Effectiveness and moderating variables. *Clinical Child and Family Psychology Review, 11*(3), 114.

Nwabuzor Ogbonnaya, I., Martin, J., & Walsh, C. R. (2018). Using the California Evidence-Based Clearinghouse for Child Welfare as a Tool for Teaching Evidence-Based Practice. *Journal of Social Work Education, 54*(sup1), S31–S40.

Oka, M., & Whiting, J. (2013). Bridging the clinician/researcher gap with systemic research: The case for process research, dyadic, and sequential analysis. *Journal of Marital and Family Therapy, 39*(1), 17–27.

Otto, H. U., Polutta, A., & Ziegler, H. (2009). Reflexive professionalism as a second generation of evidence-based practice: Some considerations on the special issue "What works? Modernizing the knowledge-base of social work". *Research on Social Work Practice, 19*, 472–478.

Owenz, M., & Hall, S. R. (2011). Bridging the research-practice gap in psychotherapy training: Qualitative analysis of master's students' experiences in a student-led research and practice team. *North American Journal of Psychology, 13*(1).

Parrish, D. E., & Rubin, A. (2012). Social workers' orientations toward the evidence-based practice process: A comparison with psychologists and licensed marriage and family therapists. *Social Work, 57*(3), 201–210.

Parker, E. O., Chang, J., & Thomas, V. (2016). A content analysis of quantitative research in journal of marital and family therapy: A 10-year review. *Journal of Marital and Family Therapy, 42*(1), 3–18.

Pinsof, W., & Wynne, L. (Eds.). (1995). Special issue: The effectiveness of marital and family therapy. *Journal of Marital and Family Therapy, 21*(4).

Powell, B. J., McMillen, J. C., Proctor, E. K., Carpenter, C. R., Griffey, R. T., Bunger, A. C., ... & York, J. L. (2012). A compilation of strategies for implementing clinical innovations in health and mental health. *Medical Care Research and Review, 69*(2), 123-157.

Powell, B. J., Waltz, T. J., Chinman, M. J., Damschroder, L. J., Smith, J. L., Matthieu, M. M., ... & Kirchner, J. E. (2015). A refined compilation of implementation strategies: Results from the Expert Recommendations for Implementing Change (ERIC) project. *Implementation Science, 10*(1), 21.

Proctor, E. K. (2007). Implementing evidence-based practice in social work education: Principles, strategies, and partnerships. *Research on Social Work Practice, 17*(5), 583–591.

Proctor, E., Silmere, H., Raghavan, R., Hovmand, P., Aarons, G., Bunger, A., ... & Hensley, M. (2011). Outcomes for implementation research: Conceptual distinctions, measurement challenges, and research agenda. *Administration and Policy in Mental Health and Mental Health Services Research, 38*(2), 65-76.

Raimy, V. (Ed.). (1950). *Training in clinical psychology*. Prentice-Hall.

Reitman, D., & McMahon, R. J. (2013). Constance "Connie" Hanf (1917–2002): The mentor and the model. *Cognitive and Behavioral Practice, 20*(1), 106–116.

Rubin, A. (2007). Improving the teaching of evidence-based practice: Introduction to the special issue. *Research on Social Work Practice, 17*(5), 541–547.

Rubin, A., & Parrish, D. (2007). Views of evidence-based practice among faculty in master of social work programs: A national survey. *Research on Social Work Practice, 17*(1), 110–122.

Sackett, D. L., Rosenberg, W. M., Gray, J. M., Haynes, R. B., & Richardson, W. S. (1996). Evidence based medicine: What it is and what it isn't. *Clinical Orthopaedics and Related Research, 455*, 3–5.

Sackett, D. L. (1997). February). *Evidence-based medicine. Seminars in Perinatology, 21*(1), 3–5.

Sanders, M. R. (1999). Triple P-Positive Parenting Program: Towards an empirically validated multilevel parenting and family support strategy for the prevention of behavior and emotional problems in children. *Clinical Child and Family Psychology Review, 2*(2), 71–90.

Saxe, G. N., Ellis, B. H., & Kaplow, J. B. (2007). *Collaborative treatment of traumatized children and teens: The trauma systems therapy approach.* Guilford Press.

Schoenwald, S. K., Sheidow, A. J., & Letourneau, E. J. (2004). Toward effective quality assurance in evidence-based practice: Links between expert consultation, therapist fidelity, and child outcomes. *Journal of Clinical Child and Adolescent Psychology, 33*(1), 94–104.

Schoenwald, S. K. (2011). It's a bird, it's a plane, it's... fidelity measurement in the real world. *Clinical Psychology: Science and Practice, 18*(2), 142–147.

Scott, K., & Lewis, C. C. (2015). Using measurement-based care to enhance any treatment. *Cognitive and Behavioral Practice, 22*(1), 49–59.

Sexton, T., & Turner, C. W. (2011). The effectiveness of functional family therapy for youth with behavioral problems in a community practice setting. *Couple and Family Psychology: Research and Practice, 1*(S), 3–15.

Shadish, W. R., Ragsdale, K., Glaser, R. R., & Montgomery, L. M. (1995). The efficacy and effectiveness of marital and family therapy: A perspective from meta-analysis. *Journal of Marital and Family Therapy, 21*(4), 345–360.

Sholomaskas, D. E., Syracuse-Siewert, G., Rounsaville, B. J., Ball, S. A., Nuro, K. F., & Carroll, K. M. (2005). We don't train in vain: A dissemination trial of three strategies of training clinicians in cognitive-behavioral therapy. *Journal of Consulting and Clinical Psychology, 73* (1), 106–115.

Silverman, W. K., & Hinshaw, S. P. (2008). The second special issue on evidence-based psychosocial treatments for children and adolescents: A 10-year update. *Journal of Clinical Child and Adolescent Psychology, 37*, 1–7.

Smith-Boydston, J. M., Holtzman, R. J., & Roberts, M. C. (2014). Transportability of Multisystemic Therapy to community settings: Can a program sustain outcomes without MST services oversight? *Child & Youth Care Forum, 43*(5), 593–605.

Sparks, J. A., & Muro, M. L. (2009). Client-directed wraparound: The client as connector in community collaboration. *Journal of Systemic Therapies, 28*, 63–76.

Straus, S. E., Glasziou, P., Richardson, W. S., & Haynes, R. B. (2011). *Evidence-based medicine: How to practice and teach it* (4th ed.). New York, NY: Churchill Livingstone.

Straus, S. E., & McAlister, F. A. (2000). Evidence-based medicine: a commentary on common criticisms. *Canadian Medical Association Journal, 163*(7), 837–841.

Sue, S., Zane, N., Nagayama Hall, G. C., & Berger, L. K. (2009). The case for cultural competency in psychotherapeutic interventions. *Annual Review of Psychology, 60*, 525–548.

Strifler, L., Cardoso, R., McGowan, J., Cogo, E., Nincic, V., Khan, P. A., ... & Treister, V. (2018). Scoping review identifies significant number of knowledge translation theories, models, and frameworks with limited use. *Journal of Clinical Epidemiology, 100*, 92-102.

Suter, J. C., & Bruns, E. J. (2008). A narrative review of wraparound outcome studies. *Resource guide to wraparound.* Portland, OR: National Wraparound Initiative, Research and Training Center for Family Support and Children's Mental Health.

Stith, S. M. (2014). What does this mean for graduate education in marriage and family therapy? commentary on "The divide between 'evidenced–based' approaches and practitioners of traditional theories of family therapy". *Journal of Marital and Family Therapy, 40*(1), 17–19.

Swenson, C. C., Schaeffer, C. M., Henggeler, S. W., Faldowski, R., & Mayhew, A. M. (2010). Multisystemic therapy for child abuse and neglect: A randomized effectiveness trial. *Journal of Family Psychology, 24*, 497–507.

Tabak, R. G., Khoong, E. C., Chambers, D. A., & Brownson, R. C. (2012). Bridging research and practice: Models for dissemination and implementation research. *American Journal of Preventive Medicine, 43*(3), 337–350.

Tan, K. M. (2002). Influence of educational outreach visits on behavioral change in health professionals. *Journal of Continuing Education in the Health Professions, 22*(2), 122–124.

Thyer, B. (2013). Evidence-based practice or evidence-guided practice: A rose by any other name would smell as sweet [Invited response to Gitterman & Knight's "Evidence-guided practice"]. *Families in Society: The Journal of Contemporary Social Services, 94*(2), 79–84.

Thyer, B. A., & Myers, L. L. (2011). The quest for evidence-based practice: A view from the United States. *Journal of Social Work, 11,* 8–25.

Thyer, B. A., & Pignotti, M. (2016). The problem of pseudoscience in social work continuing education. *Journal of Social Work Education, 52*(2), 136–146.

Trupin, E. J., Kerns, S. E. U., Walker, S. C., DeRobertis, M. T., & Stewart, D. G. (2011). Family integrated transitions: A promising program for juvenile offenders with co-occurring disorders. *Journal of Child & Adolescent Substance Abuse, 20*(5), 421–436.

Walker, J. S., & Bruns, E. J. (2006). Building on practice-based evidence: Using expert perspectives to define the wraparound process. *Psychiatric Services, 57*(11), 1579–1585.

Wampold, B. (2001). *The great psychotherapy debate.* Mahwah, NJ: Lawrence Erlbaum.

Wampold, B. E., & Bhati, K. S. (2004). Attending to the omissions: A historical examination of evidence-based practice movements. *Professional Psychology: Research and Practice, 35,* 563–570.

Wandersman, A., Imm, P., Chinman, M., & Kaftarian, S. (2000). Getting to outcomes: A results-based approach to accountability. *Evaluation and Program Planning, 23*(3), 389–395.

Washington State Institute for Public Policy and University of Washington Evidence Based Practices Institute. (2012). *Inventory of evidence-based, research-based, and promising practices.* Report ID: E2SHB2536.

Washington State Institute for Public Policy and University of Washington Evidence Based Practices Institute. (2014). *Updated inventory of evidence-based, research-based, and promising practices for prevention and intervention services for children and juveniles in child welfare, juvenile justice, and mental health systems.* Report ID: E2SHB2536-5.

Waters, T., Marzano, R. J., & McNulty, B. (2003). Balanced leadership: What 30 years of research tells us about the effect of leadership on student achievement. A working paper. Retrieved from https://eric.ed.gov/?id=ED481972.

Webb, S. A. (2001). Some considerations on the validity of evidence-based practice in social work. *British Journal of Social Work, 31*(1), 57–79.

Webster-Stratton, C., & Reid, M. J. (2003). The incredible years parents, teachers and children training series: A multifaceted treatment approach for young children with conduct problems. In J. R. Weisz, & A. E. Kazdin, (Eds.). *Evidence-based psychotherapies for children and adolescents.* (3rd ed.), 194-210.

Weisz, J. R., Kuppens, S., Eckshtain, D., Ugueto, A. M., Hawley, K. M., & Jensen-Doss, A. (2013). Performance of evidence-based youth psychotherapies compared with usual clinical care: A multilevel meta-analysis. *JAMA Psychiatry, 70,* 750–761.

Weisz, J. R., Moore, P. S., Southam-Gerow, M. A., Weersing, V. R., Valeri, S. M., & McCarty, C. A. (2005). *Therapist's manual PASCET: Primary and secondary control enhancement training program.* Los Angeles, CA: University of California.

Wisdom, J. P., Chor, K. H. B., Hoagwood, K. E., & Horwitz, S. M. (2014). Innovation adoption: A review of theories and constructs. *Administration and Policy in Mental Health and Mental Health Services Research, 41*(4), 480–502.

Zlotnik, J. (2007). Evidence-based practice and social work education: A view from Washington. *Research on Social Work Practice, 17,* 625–629.

Index

© Springer Nature Switzerland AG 2019
R. Bertram and S. Kerns, *Selecting and Implementing Evidence-Based Practice*,
https://doi.org/10.1007/978-3-030-11325-4